How to Develop Your Career in Dental Nursing

Janine Brooks MBE, DMedEth, MSc, FFGDP(UK), MCDH, DDPHRCS, BDS, FAcadMEd

CEO of Dentalia Coaching and Training Consultancy, co-founder of Dental Mentors UK and registration assessment panellist for the General Dental Council

Fiona Ellwood BEM, MEd LM, PG Cert HF/E, PG Cert PH, PG Cert DMent, BA (Hons) Ed S, (Hon) FFGDP, former FDTF RCS (Ed), MAadMEd, NSCTS practitioner, mental health first aider

Specialist expert advisor at Bangor University, education associate and registration panel member for the General Dental Council

WILEY Blackwell

Registered Offices
John Wiley & Sons, Inc., 111 River Street, Hoboken, NJ 07030, USA
John Wiley & Sons Ltd, The Atrium, Southern Gate, Chichester, West Sussex, PO19 8SQ, UK

For details of our global editorial offices, customer services, and more information about Wiley products visit us at www.wiley.com.

Wiley also publishes its books in a variety of electronic formats and by print-on-demand. Some content that appears in standard print versions of this book may not be available in other formats.

Library of Congress Cataloging-in-Publication Data applied for
ISBN: 9781119861706; ePDF: 9781119861713; epub: 9781119861720; oBook: 9781119861737

Cover Design: Wiley
Cover Image: © Feodora/Adobe Stock Photos

Set in 10.5/13pt Minion by Straive, Pondicherry, India
Printed and bound by CPI Group (UK) Ltd, Croydon, CR0 4YY

C9781119861706_120523

How to
Develop
Your Career
in Dental Nursing

'. . . We shall not cease from exploration
And the end of all our exploring
Will be to arrive where we started
And know the place for the first time.'

T.S Eliot (1888–1965)

Dedication

To all those early dental nurses who paved the way for today.
To all the dental nurses of today who are paving the way for
the future of the profession. Be proud.

Contents

About the authors

Fiona Ellwood BEM

General Dental Council registrant and mental health wellness campaigner

MEd LM, PG Cert HF/E, PG Cert Public Health, PG Cert Mentoring in Dentistry, BA (Hons) Ed S, PG Cert Ed (PGCE), (Hon) FFGDP (UK), FDTF (RCS Ed) IAM and RSPH fellowships, NCSCT practitioner, doctoral student, trustee of Dentaid

Fiona is a member of the Executive Board and elected President 2019–22 of the Society of British Dental Nurses, leading on Education Governance and Quality Assurance with a special interest in public health matters. She is the Immediate Past Chair of the National Oral Health Promotion Group and is a key opinion leader and an advisor. She writes extensively for a number of journals. Fiona has been a dental nurse for 37 years, although she first entered the field 40 years ago. She speaks nationally and internationally on related topics. She is immensely proud to have been involved in the Scottish Dental Clinical Effectiveness Programme (SDCEP) research during the pandemic and many key stakeholder meetings.

Fiona is a trained and practising mentor and mental health first aider, with many years of experience. She has studied and been successful at Masters level and is a doctorate student. She is a subject expert at Bangor University, Wales, and part of the innovative work that is rethinking and redesigning dental education and training. Fiona is an external examiner in the Republic of Ireland and is a member of the Human Factors Advisory Board. She is co-chairing a four-nation mental health wellness framework for adoption in primary and secondary care, across all dental professional groups, having gained the support of chief dental officers and the Royal Colleges, as well as the regulators.

In 2019 Fiona was appointed to the Interim Education Advisors Board, RCS Edinburgh, and represents the Dental Dean on the One Voice work; she is also a regional ambassador for RCS Edinburgh. She was the first dental care professional to receive an honorary fellowship from the FGDP (UK) RCS England and one of the first to be awarded the fellowship of the Faculty of Dental Trainers, RCS Edinburgh. Fiona was also privileged to be appointed the (Hon) Vice President of the British Society of Dental Hygiene and Therapy (BSDHT). Fiona is a former President of the British Association of Dental Nurses and an examiner for the National Examining Board of Dental Nurses and the Oral Health Education Examining Board.

Fiona is an education associate for the GDC and a member of the Registration Panel; she has also advised for Quality and Qualifications Ireland (QQI) Republic of Ireland. She is a trustee at Dentaid and supports the Mouth Cancer Foundation on education matters. To this end, she has also been working on an implementation programme for sustainable oral health in Nepal via RCS Edinburgh. Fiona has been instrumental in setting up the Dental Professional Alliance, a group where all dental care professional presidents meet to discuss matters of interest and to work together when the need arises. She is also proud to have brought to fruition the 'SafeSpace' initiative for dental nurse students.

In June 2019 Fiona was awarded the British Empire Medal in the Queen's Birthday Honours for her contribution to dentistry. On 12 March 2021, Fiona was very proud to co-announce the launch of the International Federation of Dental Assistants and Nurses in which she, on behalf of the Society of British Dental Nurses, has played an instrumental part.

In 2021 she was presented with an award from the NEBDN for her contribution to dental nurse education and spoke on advocacy for the British Fluoridation Society. Fiona is currently a co-investigator as part of an NIHR research project with Newcastle University.

Dr Janine Brooks MBE

DMed Eth, MSc, FFGDP(UK), MCDH, DDPH(RCS), BDS, FAcadMEd, CEO of Dentalia Coaching and Training Consultancy, Director of the Dental Coaching Academy, co-founder of Dental

Mentors UK, private coach and mentor (Remediation, Career and Personal Development), registration assessment panellist for the General Dental Council, trustee of the Dentists' Health Support Trust, expert witness, trustee of the NHS Retirement Fellowship and honorary fellow, Society of British Dental Nurses.

Janine enjoys a portfolio career working across a number of roles and organisations. Themes running through her work include education, mentoring and coaching. She launched her own coaching and training consultancy, Dentalia, in July 2011, providing coaching and mentoring to dental professionals and a broad range of education and training topics. She writes extensively and has published several books, plus a number of articles and papers over the years.

Janine qualified from University of Birmingham dental school in 1983 and spent 19 years working as a community dentist in Herefordshire and Warwickshire before taking on national roles. She has Masters degrees in community dental health and health informatics and a doctorate in medical ethics. Since 2011 she has been a sole trader and has enjoyed expanding her portfolio of work. Her main interests lie in bio-ethics, professionalism, leadership in dentistry and mentoring.

Janine was thrilled to receive an MBE for services to dentistry in 2007.

Fiona and Janine share a deep interest in education and training within dentistry – their paths initially crossed whilst working with National Vocational Qualifications. The history and development of dental nursing is another area of shared interest for them.

Foreword

Janine and Fiona have set out to spotlight the development and changes in dental nursing over the last 150 years. In this book, they not only capture the history of dental nursing, they also share comparisons of progress, inside and outside the United Kingdom, and celebrate success. So often information or comment on dental nursing is integrated to texts on dentists so it was pleasing to read their 'focused' approach.

When I reflect on the detailed timelines they have constructed, I was reminded of the term 'living memory'. In the early 1980s, when I qualified, the acronym 'DSA' and the phrase 'The Girls' were common parlance in dental surgeries and practices in reference to dental team members. In my early career, I was an associate dentist in a branch practice with a young unqualified dental assistant. I turned to Fiona to help me engage this young, willing woman to train, develop and qualify. I could not believe what was involved – not only in specific clinical tasks but in background reading and knowledge. Good grounding to be involved with the Greater Manchester team organising the first course for dental nurses in England to apply fluoride varnish in Salford three decades later. Dental nurses must now be viewed and respected as assets to dentistry and patients, not just employees 'assisting with specific tasks' in surgeries. I think this book will lead readers to that conclusion.

Disease experience and patient values are changing. There is an increasing emphasis on a preventive and personalised approach to dental care provision. Why is it taking so long for dental nurses to gain career development opportunities, structure and reward in clinical posts? The authors celebrate successes. A growing number of dental nurses have progressed their careers and been appointed to senior leadership positions, often due to their experience and responsibilities outside the clinical environment. I witnessed the high regard and respect that dental nursing skills and knowledge attracted outside dentistry when some were redeployed in the COVID-19 pandemic to intensive treatment units, general wards and vaccination centres. Fiona and Janine's book reminds us that it is time for the profession as a whole to put in place measures that will allow greater opportunity for career progression within the clinical sphere of dentistry and beyond.

Fiona has worked untiringly to raise the profile of dental nurses and steer career pathways and opportunities, with many still to come. Janine has worked tirelessly on personal development, coaching and workforce development in her distinguished career. She and Fiona remind us in this book that we must learn from what has gone before. Despite the acknowledged challenges within the dental system, and in the NHS dental contracting environment in particular, there are no two people better placed than the authors to take the 'how to do it' discussion on career progression, respect and reward for clinical dental nurses forward. I agree with their assumption that dental nurses who qualify in 2023 will be very different from dental nurses who are about to retire. I look forward to the sequel to this book!

Colette Bridgman MBE
Retired Consultant in Dental Public Health
CDO Wales 2016–2021

Preface

When the idea for this book was first conceived, we wanted to write about a topic that was dear to both our hearts – dental nurses. We felt that while there were books that included dental nurses, there were few that majored on them. We were also conscious that the history of dental nurses was not always well appreciated, even by those within the profession. We are advocates for the value that dental nurses bring to the dental team and for their advancement to expand their role to undertake expanded duties.

It sometimes takes time before it's possible to write about something and both Janine and Fiona have certainly served time within dentistry. From early on in their careers, they showed their support and encouragement for the advancement of dental nurses. Fiona began working as a dental nurse back in 1979, the same year that Janine entered University of Birmingham dental school. However, it was not until 2000 that their paths crossed in Nottingham. They were both working with National Vocational Qualifications, Fiona as an internal verifier and Janine as an external verifier.

Their history of working with dental nurse qualifications goes back further than that. Janine was an examiner for the NEBDN Dental Nurse qualification from 1986. She also introduced an evening class for trainee dental nurses to prepare for their examination. She taught on the course and guided about 50 dental nurses to successful completion. She continued her interest with dental nurse education when she was part of the team who developed and introduced the Foundation Degree for Dental Nursing at the University of Northampton. For about 20 years Janine worked clinically in community dentistry, treating special needs adults and also honing her general management skills. More recently, she launched her own consultancy and training business, Dentalia, providing postqualification training and education alongside coaching and mentoring.

Fiona was a practising dental nurse in the Lake District and moved to Manchester where she eventually pursued her dental nursing career and qualification. Having completed her qualification, she began training and mentoring student dental nurses as a senior dental nurse. One student led to another and education became a key component of her work. Over the years, she has taught many dental nurses across a number of different courses and levels of qualifications, at one point running a dental nurse training business. She too was an examiner for the NEBDN for both the primary qualification and the oral health examinationm and a tutor and internal verifier for the City and Guilds programme where she took pride in supporting other dental nurses. Fiona went on to develop the Foundation Degree at Chester University and co-lead on several of the modules. Since then, Fiona has taken on mentorship roles to support dental nurses in becoming tutors and has acted as a supervisor for a number of dental nurses undertaking higher education qualifications. In 2017 Fiona joined the University of Bangor and with colleagues developed the first Welsh dental nursing qualifications, at levels 3 and 4. More recently, she has been leading projects which help dental nurses make good career choices and has acted as a facilitator for international collaboration work. Fiona has been instrumental as a founder of the Society of British Dental Nurses and a co-founder of the International Federation of Dental Assistants and Dental Nurses, always placing dental nurses at the heart of everything she does.

Both Fiona and Janine have been educational associates for the General Dental Council for a number of years, a quality assurance role working with providers of dental education and training. We have worked both clinically and in national, strategic positions, allowing us to develop a broader overview of the profession. This has greatly enlarged our personal networks, which have proved extremely useful in gathering information for the book.

We have built upon these years of experience and expert knowledge in the writing of the book. We hope it will spark an interest within readers to look more deeply at the profession of dental nursing and the potential it offers as we move into the future. This is not just a look back on important history, it is also an analysis of what we have today, in the form of opportunities for career advancement. Even more than that, we have scanned the horizon to try to open a window on the future.

We have offered a great deal of food for thought throughout the book and have an eye on the future too – there are other actors who can help to enable dental nurses to reach new heights and be the professionals that they aspire to be. We still have a long way to go and perhaps this book simply scratches the surface. However, we hope that it will be a catalyst to stimulate debate, provoke high-level discussions and ultimately bring about transformation and change.

Acknowledgements

Foremost, we would like to express our gratitude to a number of colleagues for their encouragement, guidance and insight as each chapter unfolded and without whom the chapters would have had a much narrower focus.

We would like to thank Robynn Rixse BS, CDA, EFDA, MADAA, FAADOM, CDIPC, the former president of the American Dental Assistants Association, who guided us through the world of dental assisting in America and helped to navigate the way through the comparative clinical activity and qualifications.

We would also like to thank Stephanie Kavanagh, former Executive Director of the Canadian Dental Assistants Association, for her direction and guidance as we unpicked the world of dental assisting in Canada. Additional thanks goes to both Robynn and Stephanie for their part in the evolution of the International Federation of Dental Assistants and Dental Nurses.

This book could not have been completed without the kindness of Helen Nield, Head of Library and Knowledge Services of the British Dental Association, Stanley Gelbier, emeritus professor of dental public health at King's College London, Brian Williams of the Lindsay Society and Paul Langmaid, former Chief Dental Officer of Wales and trustee of the Dentists' Health Support Trust.

A further thank you goes to all those colleagues who have answered endless questions and provided insight into their view of dentistry and dental nursing.

Finally, we would like to thank Colette Bridgman, former Chief Dental Officer of Wales and consultant in dental public health, for her generous foreword. Throughout her extensive career, she not only recognised the skills and abilities of dental nurses, but also ensured change happened and left doors open for others to continue in the same vein, as she retired in July 2021.

Chapter 1 **Introduction**

> '*The farther backward you can look, the farther forward you can see.*'
>
> Winston Churchill (Smith 2021/Winston Churchill)

What a great sentiment from Winston Churchill. We hope we can do justice to the quote as we look back on the growth of dental nursing and shine a spotlight on both the past and the present, whilst importantly pointing to the future.

Both of us have been fortunate to enjoy long careers in dentistry, Fiona as a dental nurse and Janine as a dentist. Even after 40 years, we continue to enjoy our work. Our paths first collided when we were both involved in National Vocational Qualifications (NVQ) and since then we have often found ourselves working on similar aspects of dentistry. It has been a pleasure working together to write this book and we both feel it is important to bring together the history of dental nursing, both ancient and modern. Building on the history, we discuss the modern landscape of dental nursing and bring in a flavour of the profession across the globe. We hope we can speak to an interest within the reader for this important and sometimes less well-covered member of the dental family.

We aim to explore the history, current position and possible futures for individual dental nurses and the profession of dental nursing within dentistry in the UK and worldwide. Social and gender considerations will be included as well as the position of dental nursing within dentistry as a whole. An important aspect will be the role of dental nursing and how this has changed over time. We hope to present a retrospective account of dental nursing over time, consolidate

How to Develop Your Career in Dental Nursing, First Edition. Edited by Janine Brooks and Fiona Ellwood.
© 2023 John Wiley & Sons Ltd. Published 2023 by John Wiley & Sons Ltd.

that into the current perspective and to open minds and thoughts in taking the profession forward into the future.

The book has been structured into seven chapters. This introductory chapter introduces the topics and issues which will be more deeply discussed in each subsequent chapter. In Chapter 2, the history of dental nursing and the dental nurse from early history to the present day will be explored. This sets the scene for the profession as we see it in the twenty-first century. Next, the current situation worldwide will be outlined and discussed. This is followed by chapters on training and qualifications; career development opportunities; followed by horizon scanning for the future. The final chapter will cover discussion and conclusions.

We are keen that the book celebrates dental nursing and recognises the considerable achievements that have been made over the past 125 years. It is true that there have been obstacles along the way and the current situation is far from perfect, but we do not want to forget that progress builds on the past. Dental nurses of the twenty-first century stand on the shoulders of those who went before.

Dental nurses, currently and historically, generally assist clinicians and have very little true clinical autonomy, but there are signs that this is changing. Since mandatory registration with the General Dental Council (GDC) in 2008, dental nurses take full responsibility for their own professionalism. They must conform to the same ethical principles as all categories of dental professional (GDC 2013). Within this book, the role of the dental nurse as we know it now and the earlier perspectives will be unveiled and the changes over the years examined. Key milestones will be highlighted with a view to the future in mind.

It is clear to see that the role and position of dental nursing has changed over time and particularly since mandatory registration was introduced in the UK. However, this is not the same for dental nurses in North America and Canada nor indeed other countries who recognise the role of the dental nurse. Change has occurred across the globe but not always in the same manner. We will highlight some of these differences in Chapter 3.

Dental nurses hold a crucial role within the dental profession and society of the UK. They are often seen by patients as the bridge between themselves and the dental surgeon. It is usually the dental nurse that greets the patient in reception and guides them into the surgery and it is the dental nurse who often walks the patient back to reception once treatment is complete. The dental nurse can find themselves the member of the team that the patient asks for clarification about treatment. Perhaps the patient is less in awe of the dental nurse and finds it easier to relate to their friendly face. That said, let there be no mistake, the 21^s century dental nurse is every bit the professional. The GDC (2013) describes dental nurses as 'Registered dental professionals who provide clinical and other support to registrants and patients'.

Dental nursing has undergone seismic changes and developments over the last 125 years. Professional status is relatively new – it has only been since 30 July 2008 that all qualified UK dental nurses must be registered with the GDC. This meant that dental nurses, once qualified, needed to register with their professional body to be able to practise. They were now bound by the same professional requirements as dentists, dental hygienists and dental therapists. This was the final formal recognition of professional status. The Scope of Practice (GDC 2013) was introduced following the Dentists Act (Amendment) Order 2005 (HM Government 2005). This allowed dental nurses to use a wider range of skills as part of their extended duties.

The role of dental nursing has expanded over time and career opportunities have opened up. Whilst the majority of dental nurses work chairside in primary care providing patient and clinical support, dental nurses are found in a vast array of roles and environments. The role models available are no longer restricted to dental hygienist, dental therapist or indeed the dental surgeon; today, there are some truly inspirational dental nurse role models. Development can be found in clinical specialty, managerial, political, educational and national strategic positions. Career opportunities will be covered in greater detail in Chapter 5.

Over the years, the role and responsibilities of the dental nurse have evolved. When thinking about the evolution of the role, it is important to consider the various terms and compilations that have been applied as a title over the years. Of equal interest is the commonalities of these titles across nations and countries, as well as their disparateness. It is fascinating to consider the factors that underpin the development of dental nursing across the globe. These will include geography, levels of oral disease, the development of dentists and other categories of dental profession and the economic situation of individual countries. The term most commonly and synonymously applied, both historically and currently, is dental assistant.

Although there is general mention of dental assistants in England in 1909, the UK census returns show that dental nurses and dental assistants were formally recognised as being within the dental workforce as early as 1881. However, there is little written information relating to dental assistants in the UK until 1940. Early dental assistants/dental nurses in England appeared to undertake mainly administrative and chaperone roles.

The primary role of the dental assistant has been identified historically by many as assisting the dentist. What is clear is that not every dentist worked with a dental assistant and their education and training appear to have been poles apart. This is still the case in some countries. In addition, not all countries recognise being a dental assistant as a professional role. In many countries, there is minimal regulation around dental activity, and few countries articulate that dental assistants must undertake formal training, with fewer still insisting on dental assistants being formally registered with a dental regulator.

For many years in the UK, dental nurses, unlike their clinical team members, were not legally required to undertake a formal qualification or be registered in order to work in dentistry. A national qualification was available via the National Examination Board for Dental Nurses (NEBDN). In addition, there was a voluntary register for qualified dental nurses. This register was maintained by the British Nurses Standards and Training Advisory Board. The move towards qualification and registration began in 1998 when the GDC set up the Dental Auxiliaries Review Board (DARG) (GDC 1998). This review group recommended that all dental auxiliaries should be qualified and registered with the GDC. Three years later in 2001, the GDC made it known that they would seek legislation to allow statutory or compulsory registration of all professionals complementary to dentistry (PCD); this included dental nurses and dental technicians (GDC 2001). A new NVQ would be introduced in Oral Health Care Dental Nursing in 2000.

From the early days of assisting in dentistry, those who assisted received instruction and 'training' on the job from the dental surgeon with whom they worked. There was no formal education and the training would have been very practically focused and tailored to the needs of specific practices and individual dentists. It was thought that assistants did not need to understand the process of tooth decay, gum disease or the composition of the materials they mixed. They were there to assist at the chair side and to be complementary to the dental surgeon.

This began to change in the 1930s in the UK. There were two reports in the 1940s that appreciated the value a trained assistant contributed to patient care and the smooth operation of providing dentistry (Teviot Report 1946, BDA 1948). Nothing more was heard until 1993, almost 50 years later, when the Nuffield Foundation (Hancock 1993) suggested that the work of dental nurses should be 'formally reappraised, defined and nationally recognised both inside and outside dentistry'. This made three reports recommending the formal education and training of dental nurses. The tide was turning away from informal schooling by dental surgeons to formal, standard qualifications.

A survey undertaken in June 2001 found that 60% of dental nurses in Oxfordshire had no formal qualifications and only half of these nurses were currently on a training course or planning to apply for one (John et al. 2002). At that time, there were concerns that bringing in mandatory training and qualifications would undermine recruitment of dental nurses. It may be that a recognition of a thirst for knowledge by many dental nurses went unappreciated.

The British Dental Nurses and Assistants Society was formed in 1940 in Leyland, Lancashire, by dental nurse Madeleine (Bunty) Winter and dentist P.E. Grundy. Bunty, as she was known, was the Association's first General Secretary in the early 1940s. In 1943, the Association held the first dental nurse examination and Bunty Winter was one of the first dental nurses to become qualified. Only dentists were allowed to be examiners until 1978 when senior nurses were also accepted onto the Board. The resulting Examination Board for Dental Nurses and Assistants remained part of the Association until 1988, when it became a separate organisation. The Association set up a voluntary register in the 1960s and became a trade union in the 1970s. From their first inception, with the exception of dental technology, non-dentist dental professional roles have been the majority preserve of women. This is another tide that began to turn from the 1980s onwards.

The numbers of PCDs steadily increased after the 1921 Dentists' Act but it was during the Second World War that PCDs became properly organised.

The future is a mixture of progression of what we know today mixed with developments, some predictable and others completely novel. If you think back over your own career since you first entered dentistry, you get a flavour of the predictable and the totally unknown. In Chapter 6, we have included an image of our own careers to illustrate this point. In many ways, preparation for the future is a combination of taking opportunities as they present and broadening experience, but even more important is keeping an open, flexible attitude and not closing off too many avenues. A growth mindset, as we will discuss, is perhaps the most valuable asset you can develop.

As we will demonstrate, dental nurses in the UK have risen from being the chaperone and the person who mixed materials and cleaned the surgery to a vital member of the dental team. They are essential to the smooth and safe provision of patient care in the dental environments of the twenty-first century.

Since the end of the twentieth century, professional ethics and society have moved away from a paternalistic approach, where the professional knew best and the patient acquiesced to their superior knowledge and expertise, toward a patient-centred approach. Partnership working with patients, where they are more fully engaged in their care, has taken centre stage. This has been accompanied by the need to ensure that dentistry employs an evidence-based approach to treatments and interventions. Both patient-centred care and evidence base require an emphasis on communication with patients. This is often an area where dental nurses excel.

As we have researched for the book and consulted with many people, we realise there will be aspects that we have only briefly covered and topics left untouched. Our apologies for those deficiencies – we have tried to give as wide a coverage as possible, knowing we may have fallen short of our target. However, if we have opened the door to others wanting to know more and encouraged you to dig a little deeper, then we have succeeded.

Note

Census data have been taken from the 'Find my past' website: www.findmypast.co.uk. This is a subscription genealogical database. Records of UK census returns from 1841 to 1921 can be searched on line.

References

British Dental Association, Incorporated Dental Society and Public Dental Service Association (1948). *Report of the Review of the Committee of Enquiry into the Training, Wages, Conditions of Service and Title of Women Assisting Dentists in Public and Private Dental Service*. British Dental Association, London.

General Dental Council (1998). Professionals Complementary to Dentistry: A consultation paper. Available at: www.gdc-uk.org

General Dental Council (2001). Summary of Council decisions taken. Available at: www.gdc-uk.org

General Dental Council (2013). Scope of Practice (updated 2019). Available at: www.gdc-uk.org

HM Government (2005). Dentist Act 1984 (Amendment) Order 2005. Available at: www.legislation.gov.uk

Hancock, R. (1993). *Education and Training of Personnel Auxiliary to Dentistry*. Nuffield Foundation, London.

John, J.H., Thomas, D., Richards, D., Evans, C. (2002). Regulating dental nursing in the UK. *BDJ*, **199**, 207–209.

Smith, D. (2021). *100 Inspirational Quotes by Winston Churchill*. Independently published.

Teviot Report (1946). *Final Report of the Inter-departmental Committee on Dentistry* (Cmd 6727). National Archives, London. Available at: www.nationalarchives.gov.uk/

Chapter 2   Early history of dental nursing

Before exploring the field and the roles of dental nursing as we know it today, it is important to take a deep dive into the historical beginnings which have shaped the current dental nursing landscape. Looking at history is an important part of planning for the future. If we are unaware of history, we could fail to build upon what went before or we could duplicate work already done. History is easy to forget but we do so at our peril.

In this chapter, we describe and analyse the role of the dental nurse throughout history, looking at how the assistant in the dental surgery first emerged and how the role has developed over the years to become the profession we know in the twenty-first century. The chapter will include an exploration of gender and, in particular, the role of women and how that has been affected by equality reforms and changes in the profession and society. Research on the history of dental nursing is not common, but it is possible to make interesting connections with the history of general nursing which has been much more widely reported.

Understanding where a profession comes from is important in order to determine what it is today and where it is going tomorrow. Knowing the history helps to put into context current issues, for example cultural and social influences. Having that knowledge fosters professional identity and a pride in how those who have assisted dental operators have contributed to the care of patients.

Ailments of the teeth, gums and soft tissues of the mouth have been endured by most hominin species and probably for hundreds of thousands of years. Tooth wear in the form of dental erosion and abrasion has been found in fossilised teeth of *Australopithecus africanus*

How to Develop Your Career in Dental Nursing, First Edition. Edited by
Janine Brooks and Fiona Ellwood.
© 2023 John Wiley & Sons Ltd. Published 2023 by John Wiley & Sons Ltd.

(Benazzi et al. 2013). Dental caries has been noted in teeth of ancient humans (Fuss et al. 2018). Traces of periodontal disease have been found in the remains of ancient Egyptians (Forshaw 2009a). Interestingly, our Romano-British ancestors may have suffered less periodontal disease than we do today (Raitapuro-Murray et al. 2014).

Individuals who ministered to and attempted to alleviate dental and oral ailments have probably also been around for a very long time. What is almost certain is that people with skill in helping to reduce the pain and discomfort of oral ailments have existed for thousands of years, so people who assisted them will also have existed – by whatever name they chose to identify themselves. Who knows what words were used to describe those individuals? However, we do know that modern dental professionals have been working in society for a relatively short time.

Dentistry appears to have entered our understanding of history a few thousand years ago with the earliest recording of a dentist to be found in Egypt. About 2660 BC, a dentist by the name of Hesyre is known from his tomb at Saqqara, close to Cairo (Forshaw 2013). Hesyre was multi-talented – he was known as the chief of dentists and the chief of physicians at the time of his death. Not only known for his healthcare, he also held a number of other religious and secular positions. Probably at the time it was the norm for a person to perform several roles, particularly combining dental and medical duties. Clearly, if Hesyre was chief of dentists, he will not have been alone, nor would he have sprung up as the first. However, his predecessors remain unknown, to date.

It may be that those who practised what we would call dentistry were not that many. Forshaw (2009b) reviewed the presence of dentistry in ancient Egypt. He looked at a range of evidence including hieroglyphic inscriptions and the dentitions of mummified and skeletal remains. He also reviewed ancient documents and artefacts. In his conclusions he notes: 'Operative dental treatment, if it did exist at all, was extremely limited'. In the hieroglyphic inscriptions that Forshaw examined, he found 150 inscriptions stating that the person depicted had medical connections, nine of which noted the person to be a dentist. Those nine individuals were described in a number of ways including; 'one who is concerned with teeth' and 'one who deals with teeth'. There was also recognition of 'chief of dentists' and 'chief dentist of the palace'. It seems that people who were deemed to work with conditions of the mouth did exist in Egypt, some holding positions of authority and serving important members of society. What we cannot determine is if they worked by themselves or if they worked with assistants (those we would call dental nurses today).

Table 2.1 highlights a few of the major influences on dentistry prior to the twentieth century. We know that some early dental operators worked with an assistant, but references to such people are not formally recorded before the 1881 census (www.findmypast.co.uk).

The definition of dentistry has relevance for when society accepts the practice of dentistry as becoming established. Early 'carers' are likely to have removed painful and troublesome teeth, whilst the restoration of form and function came later.

The gender of those taking on a caring role is interesting. Although the division is not total and there remains a fuzzy boundary between the genders in the twenty-first century, currently the majority of dental

Table 2.1 Highlights in the history of dentistry.

Date	Group/individual	Event
3000–2151 BC	Egyptians	Hesyre is the earliest dentist known by name
900–300 BC	Mayans	Teeth receive attention for religious reasons or self-adornment
460–322 BC	Greeks	Hippocrates and Aristotle write about tooth decay
166–201 AD	Romans	Restore decayed teeth with gold crowns
570–950	Muslims	Use Siwak as a primitive toothbrush
1510–1590	Ambroise Paré	Writes extensively about dentistry, including extractions
1678–1761	Pierre Fauchard	'Father of modern dentistry'
1728–1793	John Hunter	Performs first scientific study of teeth
1844	Horace Wells	Uses nitrous oxide for relief of dental pain
1881	Miss Fanny Payne	First dental nurse recorded in 1881 UK census
1895	G.V. Black	Becomes 'grand old man of dentistry' and perfects amalgam

Source: pocket dentistry.com

nurses across all countries are female. Those who assisted dental surgeons in the past, however, may have been predominantly male; they were generally considered to be learning the trade and preparing to become a dentist. In that respect, they cannot truly be considered to be dental nurses – they are more likely to have been dentist apprentices. This is not a statement that can be accurately tested as records of specific dental professionals are not easy to find. A look at art depicting dental surgeons and their assistants does tend to show the assistant as male. As we move through the years, the number of females occupying the post of dental assistant or dental nurse begins to increase.

It is difficult to find references to dental nursing in its earliest forms. Dentistry in art, however, can provide some clues. One such piece of art, a print by Edward Dighton (c.1752–1819). was published in 'Some Alnwick caricatures' (1812–1817) by William Davison of Alnwick, Northumberland. The print depicts an itinerant tooth drawer, who is accompanied by his (male) assistant. The assistant, dressed in a clown's costume, is providing entertainment and distraction whilst an extraction is being undertaken. Another print by Edward Dighton, also published by William Davison, shows a village smithy. His assistant is standing on a stool supporting the patient's head against his chest. Yet another print by Edward Dighton depicts a town tooth drawer in a wealthy-looking house although it's not clear if this is the tooth drawer's house or perhaps he has made a home visit. He is accompanied by an assistant (again male) who is carrying an instrument case. Both the tooth drawer and assistant are dressed (and wigged) as wealthy individuals.

It seems we have a theme in this small selection of art by the same artist; there is an assistant but they are always male. Perhaps this says more about the position of working women in society during the late sixteenth and early seventeenth centuries. An important point is that the prints do give us evidence that dental assistants, the forerunners of dental nurses, were to be found at this time; their gender is of less importance.

We can find evidence of the dental assistant in an even earlier piece of art. A copper engraving by Lucas van Leyden, *The Dentist*, crafted in 1523, depicts a dentist at work. It appears he is operating with his assistant, a woman. Sadly, the assistant is shown placing her hand in the patient's pocket, not the greatest illustration of a dental nurse.

Dental nurses in times gone by, as today, were part of general society and in particular how society viewed women and their contribution to the wider population over time. Looking back into history, we find the philosopher Aristotle sharing his views in his book On the Generation of Animals, written in the fourth century BC (Platt 2015). He writes: 'We must look upon the female character as being a sort of natural deficiency'. Oh dear, not the best recommendation for women. One might wonder how his mother felt about her son's views.

Mortimer (2009), in his excellent book The Time Traveller's Guide to Medieval England, notes that in the twenty-first century we have come some way from the manner in which women were described in medieval times. Then, women fell into four groups: maidens, wives, nuns and widows. At that time, only widows and aged spinsters (old maids) had a degree of independence. Women were blamed for society's weakness, whether that be physical, intellectual or moral. This seems to stem from the story of Adam and Eve, when Eve tempts Adam to eat from the forbidden fruit, resulting in their fall from Eden – as Mortimer (2009) writes, 'a difficult thing to live down'. Society at that time was misogynistic to say the least. The male-dominated society was regarded as the natural way, and the position of women was believed to be a punishment from God. Maybe a convenient way to control half the population? It's always good to have someone to blame.

For a long time in the UK, women were expected to focus on their homes, their children and particularly on the unquestioning support of their husbands. Being outspoken and trying to buck the system was not only frowned upon, it could also be dangerous. Vocal unmarried women risked becoming targets of the witch hunts and being burned at the stake. Until the eighteenth century, academic education for women, particularly for women of lower socio-economic class, was uncommon and positively discouraged, as it was considered that learning would diminish the innocence of women (Purvis 1991, Symes 1995).

The nineteenth century

During the nineteenth century, it was generally considered that men and women occupied different places in society and undertook different areas of work. Ridley (2017) calls these 'different spheres'. Women occupied the private sphere of home and family, whilst men occupied the public sphere of work, business and politics. The latter sphere was considered to be the more important of the two. Not surprisingly, this meant that men were able to lead and control the world as they saw fit. Women could rarely operate outside the control of a man, whether that be father, husband or brother. This had a direct and generally limiting effect on the type of work that a woman could undertake. Once a woman was married, she was mostly confined to running the home and raising children. However, it is interesting that a small proportion of those noted in the various census returns were married, as we shall see later.

In this century, women could be found working as doctors, lawyers, in the church and teaching as well as writers and singers. However, it was not the case across the socio-economic classes. At this time, working-class women were generally working in factories or the domestic sphere.

Most working-class women in Victorian England had no choice but to work in order to help support their families. They worked in factories, in domestic service for richer households or in family businesses. Many women also carried out home-based work such as finishing garments and shoes for factories, laundry or preparation of snacks to sell in the market or streets. This was in addition to their unpaid work at home which included cooking, cleaning, childcare and often keeping small animals and growing vegetables and fruit to help feed their families.

However, women's work has not always been accurately recorded within sources that historians rely on, as much of their work was irregular, home-based or within a family-run business. Women's work was often not included in statistics on waged work in official records, altering our perspective on the work women undertook. Often women's wages were thought of as secondary earnings and less important than men's wages even though they were crucial to the family's survival. This is why the census returns from the early years of the nineteenth century often show a blank space under the occupation column against women's names – even though we now have evidence from a variety of sources from the 1850s onwards that women engaged in a wide variety of waged work in the UK.

Bullough (1994) notes that female dominance in general nursing began in the nineteenth century. The Nightingale reforms were influential and seemed to have created a stigma against men working in caring. Prior to this time, male nurses were much more numerous, particularly within the military (Ross 2017). India may have been the birthplace of nurse education (Vallano 2008) with men taking the role of nurses because of their 'pureness'. Bullough (1994) tells us that caring for the sick was not deemed to be a role that women were suited to. This may come as a surprise to us today, particularly as women totally dominate the caring professions. It would seem that Florence Nightingale flipped the gender roles for nursing and the current predominance of women as general nurses is largely due to her. Clearly, dental nurses undertake different roles from general nurses but it may be that the gender changes in general nursing had a knock-on effect for the emergence of female dental nurses.

Dental assistant duties were first formally described in the UK in 1883. At that time, those duties included arranging appointments, taking care of the office, standing at the side of the dental chair during treatment of the patient by the dentist. However, we know from the art record that dental assistants had been working in dentistry for many years before 1883. The 1881 UK census also provides evidence that at least one dental nurse was working.

It seems that when anaesthetics began to be used within dental practice after 1850, the chaperoning of women patients by women assistants became more commonplace. Their role was probably extremely limited, but it was a beginning.

Whilst the history of women in dentistry is relatively sparse, most of what is written concerns women dentists and mention of female dental nurses is particularly difficult to find. Those who undertook the role that we today know as dental nursing went under a wide variety of titles. A literature review showed the following descriptors.

Subordinate	Trained auxiliary
Lady in waiting	Chairside assistant
Dental house maiden	Dental auxiliaries
Auxiliary	Somatological assistant
Dental nurse	Dental assistant
Certified dental assistant	Registered dental assistant
Licensed dental assistant	Intraoral dental assistants
Chairside attendants	Dental dresser
Dental surgery attendant	Sick berth attendant
	to dental surgeons

Clearly, it was many years before the title became more standardised, although even this has only taken place very recently. Gelbier (2005) confirms that the title 'dental nurse' was not a new title born in the 1940s, a fact borne out by census returns, as shown in Table 2.2.

Census returns are an interesting source of information about dental nurses and dental nursing over time. Before 1918, female dentists were recognised and dental assistants were also noted within the dental environment, although at that time it was not common for dentists to work with an assistant. A review from the 1871–1939 UK census returns using the search term 'dental nurse' provided the information found in Table 2.2. The provider www.find mypast.co.uk was used for all census searches and data reproduced. Please see note at the end of the chapter.

The census of 1871 has no reported dental nurses of either gender. Ten years later, the census of 1881 shows the first dental nurse noted as an occupation in the census returns. She was Fanny Payne, single and aged 35 years. Fanny worked as a nurse at the dental hospital at St Martin in the Fields. It seems reasonable to assume that Fanny was not the only dental nurse working at the dental hospital, but there are no others recorded as such in the census return that year. In the return of 1891, two women report themselves as dental nurses, one single,

Table 2.2 UK census by year, search term 'dental nurse', by age and marital status.

Census year	Number	Gender	Age range Mean age years	Marital status
1871	0	-	-	-
1881	1	Female	35	Single
1891	2	Female	18–61	Single 1 Married 1
1901	17	Female	19–58 31	Single 15 Widowed 2
1911	71	69 Female 2 Male (both married)	17–77 29	Single 57 Widowed 7 Married 6
1921	425	406 Female 19 Male	Not available	Not available
1939	1562	1505 Female 57 Male	Not calculated	Not calculated

one married. Ann, one of those two, was 18 years old and lived in the same residence as John Wilson, a surgeon dentist. Ann is noted in the census return as a servant (nurse domestic), in relation to the head of the household, but it seems fair to assume that she was dental nurse to John Wilson. In 1911, we find the first men reporting their occupation as dental nurse. Arthur Trimnell was 41 years old, married and lived in Fulham. William Warren Alcock was 38 years old, married and worked at West Ham Borough Asylum. We find Arthur Trimnell in the 1901 census also but here his reported occupation is male nurse. We will never know if Arthur was a dental nurse in 1901 or whether he swapped from general nursing to dental nursing. Over the years, the number of recorded dental nurses begins to slowly rise and in 1921, 406 women and 19 men report themselves to be dental nurses. This number has increased to 1562 by the 1939 census.

The search becomes more interesting when the term 'dental assistant' is used. However, care must be taken in the interpretation of the term. Dental assistant is a broad umbrella title that covers those who were apprenticed to a dentist as well as those who were undertaking the role of dental nurse. In addition, it could also apply to those who worked in the dental manufacturing sector, for example technicians. Other descriptors are also found, for example dental secretary, tooth trimmer, assistant at dental depot, dental assistant moulder and dental instrument maker assistant. After 1911, the numbers become too large to accurately count individuals in each reported category. Many of the descriptors are not roles within the dental surgery. However, they are interesting as roles that women undertook within the larger remit of dentistry.

Table 2.3 shows the total number in each census year (1871–1939), denoted as dental assistants. The different role descriptors found when searching are also recorded. Only females were included in our analysis of age and marital status as it is not possible to accurately determine if the males were actually dental assistants (dental nurses) or apprentice dentists. It is appreciated that this will fail to recognise those males who were actually employed as dental assistants, specifically dental nurses. It is interesting to note that throughout the census years, there are a number of families where several children are working in the dental industry in some form or another. Sisters working in the role are particularly notable, also a small number of mothers and

Table 2.3 UK census: individuals reported as working in the dental industry 1871–1939 by age, gender and role descriptor.

Census year	Number	Gender	Role descriptors	Age range (females) years	Mean age	Marital status (females)
1871	None					–
1881	90	19 Female 71 Male	Dental Assistant	14–54	27	Single 18 Widow 1
1891	248	43 Female 205 Male	Ass. Dent. Manufacture 1 Ass. Dent. Academy 1 Dent. Works Ass. 1 Ass. Dent. Factory 1 Dental assistant 39	14–65	23	Single 41 Married 0 Widow 2
1901	447	73 Female 374 Male	Ass. Dent. Factory. 2 Ass. Dent. Depot. 2 Dent. Works ass. 8 Dent. Manufa. Ass. 1 Dental lady ass. 1 Dental assistant. 433	13–74	22	Single 72 Married 1 Widow 0
1911	809	183 Female 626 Male	Moulder's ass. Dental works Ass. Dental depot Dental lady ass. Dent. Secretary Tooth trimmer Dent. Factory ass.	17–77	29	Single 173 Married 7 Widow 3

(Continued)

Table 2.3 (Continued)

Census year	Number	Gender	Role descriptors	Age range (females) years	Mean age	Marital status (females)
			Packer at dentists			
			Dent. Manufa. Ass.			
			Dent. Instrument maker ass.			
			Dent. Acad. Ass.			
			Dent. Ass. Arti. Teeth			
			Dent. Rubber stamp ass.			
			Ass. Dental store			
			Ass. Dent. App. Dealer			
			Dent. Anaesthetist			
			Dent. Shop ass.			
			Tooth pourer ass.			
			Dent. mechanic			
1921	406 Female 19 Male		Dental Dresser (20)	Not given		
1939	1508 Female 58 Male		Dental Dresser (4)	Not analysed		

daughters. Several female dental assistants are living in the same household and, it is assumed, working for a dental surgeon who is the head of that household. Some are clearly relatives, a few are described as servants, as was the case for Ann, noted above.

The number of individuals employed as dental nurses or dental assistants grows with each census, which is not surprising as the practice of dentistry itself was growing at this time. It is clear that most of those described as dental nurses were female whilst the majority of those described as dental assistants were male. However, this is not universal but it is difficult to differentiate between the genders accurately.

The age range of those described as working within the dental sector is wide. For the three census returns between 1881 and 1901, the youngest dental nurses or dental assistants are 13–14 years, but the oldest are recorded as in their 50s, 60s and even 70s. In the census of 1911, the youngest age has risen to 17 years and the oldest 77 years. These women, whilst largely single, also include those who are married and those who are widowed. In 1881, two dental assistants are recorded as mother and daughter; the mother is a widow (at the age of 46 years). In 1891 a grandmother, mother and daughter are recorded as dental assistants; grandmother and mother are both widows (at the ages of 65 and 31 years). The grand-daughter is aged 16 years. Also, in 1891, four sets of sisters are recorded as dental assistants. In the census of 1911, 17 sets of sisters are recorded as dental assistants. The descriptor 'servant' is still used for a number of those women, who were all living in the same residence as the dentist it is presumed they worked for.

Searching the census years can reveal some interesting and tantalising pieces of information. For example, in 1871 when searching using the term 'Dental', Annie Garner is recorded. In 1871 Annie is a baby, only a few months old. She is recorded as living with her family at Soho Square Dental Hospital, St Anne, Westminster, London. Unfortunately, the occupation of her father is not recorded, so we can't know whether he was a member of staff. Soho Square Dental Hospital was the first dental school to open in Britain on 1 October 1859. It eventually became the Royal Dental Hospital in 1901.

Another interesting find came with the census of 1841 when searching using the term 'Dental'. Forty results at first looked very promising, only to find that 36 of the results were for individuals living in Dentals Street, St Leonard, Elham, Kent. A further four of the results lived in Dentals House, Borden, Milton, Kent.

In the census of 1861 three sisters are recorded with the surname De Horn, two of which were born in Australia, the youngest sister being born in Surrey, England. Why was this interesting? All the sisters have a recorded occupation of Dental co-scholar. Sadly, the exact meaning of this occupation is unknown. In the same census a female servant is included, she was born in Germany and her name was Herenerille Dental. Finally, in 1861 Sarah Ross, married aged 53 years, has a recorded occupation of Dental pupa; was she an apprentice dentist or a dental assistant?

Census returns have provided to be a fascinating source when seeking information about dental nurses. It would be interesting to undertake more research on these individuals. Who knows if a dental nurse working today is a descendant of one of these early dental nurses. However, that will have to wait for another book.

The twentieth century

UK society has experienced massive change since 1918. This includes health, wealth, technological, scientific, cultural and demographic. Men, women, young and old and at all levels of society have experienced and continue to experience the effects of that change. Women, in particular, have gained opportunities that were difficult or impossible to access prior to 1900. The changes did not happen overnight, nor all at the same time and the changes continue.

Brooks (2019) notes that the women of today may find it hard to believe the challenges experienced by their mothers, grandmothers and great-grandmothers. In the first quarter of the twenty-first century, women enjoy many freedoms that could have only been imagined by our ancestors. However, this does not mean that equality of opportunity has been achieved for all women across all areas of work. We must not forget that equality spans both genders. Males are underrepresented within dental nursing and although numbers are increasing, they constitute a very small proportion of dental nurses working today.

The end of the eighteenth century and the early part of the nineteenth century saw considerable unrest amongst many of the female and some of the male population of the UK. Ridley (2017), in her book 'Suffragettes and the Fight for the Vote', gives an excellent analysis of how some women challenged their role in society. They campaigned and fought for the right of women to vote in the UK. The suffragette movement was not confined to the UK and Great Britain was late to the party, with a number of other countries reforming their voting rights much earlier, notably New Zealand in 1893, Australia in 1902, Finland in 1906, Denmark and Iceland in 1915 (Ridley 2017).

On 6th February 1918 the Representation of the People (Equal Franchise) Act gave some women the vote as long as they were aged at least 30 and were either themselves or married to a local government elector.

Mari Takayanagi (2018, pp. 56–72) explains what this means more fully.

'*A woman had to be aged 30 or older to register as a Parliamentary voter. She, or her husband, also had to meet the local government franchise qualification, which meant:*

- *Occupying a dwelling-house (of any value). This meant living in a house or a separate part of a house, as an owner (i.e. a freehold owner) or a tenant (i.e. paying rent); or*
- *Occupying land or premises of a yearly value of not less than five pounds. This meant living as a lodger in rooms within a house, which were let in an unfurnished state. The annual value of £5 meant the gross estimated rental or gross value as assessed for rates, as determined by the registration officer.*

Therefore – living as a lodger in furnished rooms at any value, or in unfurnished rooms to a value of less than £5, did not qualify. This meant in practice women over 30 were excluded from the vote including women living at home with parents, brothers or other family members; female resident servants; and unmarried women living in furnished rooms or hostels. A woman on military or naval service in connection with the current war could vote, if she would have qualified had she not been on service, from the age of 30. A woman whose husband was on military or naval service still qualified if her husband met the local government franchise qualification.

No woman could be a conscientious objector! A woman was not disqualified from voting if her husband was a conscientious objector.

She had to be not subject to any legal incapacity, and be a British subject. If married to an alien, she was herself an alien and could not vote. Peeresses in their own right can vote!

Women had a potential second vote in the university franchise (University graduates over 21 years), but unlike men were not eligible for the business premises franchise.'

The 1918 Representation of the People (Equal Franchise) Act was a step in the right direction but only that, a step. It is likely that very few women working as dental assistants or dental nurses gained the vote at this time. To meet the age criteria, they would have had to have been born in 1888 or earlier. Once that hurdle had been achieved they (or their husband, if married) needed to be living as an owner occupier or a tenant. Living with parents or other family members did not count.

It is important to remember that the early part of the twentieth century was a period of turmoil within the UK. The First World War (1914–1918) was closely followed by the influenza pandemic and also the unrest of suffrage. These major events set the backdrop for seismic upheavals within dentistry as qualified dentists struggled to assert themselves against unqualified operators. The oral health of the population was extremely poor and the numbers of dentists (qualified or unqualified) could not meet the population need. There were some opportunities here for dental nurses and these will be explored later in the chapter.

The twentieth century was effectively a rollercoaster for dental nurses and the profession as they initially rose to undertake a wider range of duties and responsibilities. This rise proved to be short-lived. Later in the century we see the founding of dental nurse/assistant associations and formally constructed education, training and qualifications. Towards the latter quarter of the century, the preparatory work that led to registration as a stand-alone professional group within the dental family early in the twenty-first century began.

It is interesting to ponder the relationship between the oral health of the population, particularly of school children, and the increased utilisation of dental nurses. A number of factors were at play in the first half of the twentieth century including public health developments, the World Wars and the corresponding loss of male manpower plus suffrage, and eventually a more active role of government in health. A number of important Acts of Parliament also contributed to change, including the 1918 Representation of the People Act, the 1928 Representation of the People Act (Equal Suffrage) and the 1921 Dentists Act. All of these factors would affect the development of dental nursing.

Early in the century, county school boards employed county medical officers and their responsibilities included the oral health of schoolchildren. Barwise (1910) reported that 80% of children attending elementary schools in Derbyshire had carious teeth. The actual number of children affected was 72 000 of the total 90 000 in school. This was a huge problem.

Dussault (1981) gives a thorough overview of the development of the British dental profession in the first half of the twentieth century. The thesis includes a section on the Acland Report (1919) which makes illuminating reading. This was potentially an important time for dental nursing and it bears a degree of exploration as it underpins the development of the profession and the position of dental nurses in the dental family.

In 1916 the Lord President of the Privy Council appointed a Departmental Committee 'to enquire into the extent and the gravity of the evils of dental practice by persons not qualified under the Dentists' Act'. This would have been the 1878 Dentists' Act that introduced voluntary registration of dentists with the GDC. The chairman of the Committee was the Right Honorable Francis Acland. The report produced by this Committee proposed the introduction of the dental dresser, trained to perform routine operative procedures and to assist registered dentists. This was clearly a radical suggestion and judging by the response from the dental profession at the time, not a popular one.

The Acland Committee (1919) was of the opinion that: 'suitably trained and competent dental dressers or nurses acting under the effective supervision of a dentist may be usefully and safely employed in school dental work'. The British Dental Journal published a response which was largely 'wait and see'. The Representative Board of the British Dental Association (BDA) made this response to the proposals: 'The Board considers that the work suggested for dental dressers or nurses would need careful definition and efficient safeguards in the interests of the patients'. Dussault (1981, p.142) speaks of 'the fight against dental dressers (1915–1921)'.

Dr Sidney Barwise (1861–1925), the Medical Officer for Derbyshire, was the originator of the dental dresser scheme. He had previously shown himself to be particularly concerned by the oral health of schoolchildren. Barwise (1924) was of the opinion that properly trained operators could undertake simple dental procedures and this would be economically advantageous at a time when there were few dentists. It would also be an efficient way to bring simple dentistry to those who needed it, such as schoolchildren and young mothers. The simple procedures that Barwise envisaged the dental dresser undertaking included scaling and polishing, extraction of deciduous and permanent teeth and filling cavities. The BDA (Tomes 1919) was not in favour and felt the scheme to be a 'dangerous expedient'. The School Dentists supported the views of the BDA and did not support the scheme. A school dentist, in a letter to the British Dental Journal, argued that the dental dresser scheme was 'totally dangerous and impracticable'. 'A dental nurse was useful to look after the instruments and on very rare occasions to hold a child's hands'.

However, regardless of the opposition, Barwise began the training of dental dressers in 1916. Derbyshire and Birmingham became the first areas in England to set up schemes in 1917. In January 1917 Mr Charles Markham, a Chesterfield mine and steel works owner, gave £250 to Dr Barwise for the training of dental nurses to become dental dressers. The training period was not long as by May 1917, several dental dressers had been trained and began work. In Nottinghamshire, by October 1919 there were two trained dental nurses and they were learning to undertake restorations and extraction under a dentist's supervision.

It seems that the introduction of dental dressers inflamed the already delicate issue of unqualified operators providing dentistry, prior to the 1921 Act. Looking back in time from the first half of the twenty-first century, it could be considered that this was a lost opportunity to build in skill mix to the young profession of dentistry. It is interesting, however, to consider the similarity of opposing views that exist today when skill mix arguments raise their head. Dussault (1981, p.222) notes that: 'the number of authorities employing dental dressers in the early 1920s never exceeded eight and the number of dressers at work was less than thirty (BDJ 1921), the profession treated this issue as one of utmost importance and used all available political means to kill the experiment in embryo to prevent the institution of an alternative to dentists' services'. Strong words. The 1921 census return shows 20 individuals who identified as dental dressers but by 1939 this number had fallen to four.

The 1921 Dentists' Act made it mandatory for newly qualified dentists to register with the Dental Board of the UK. It also prohibited the practice of dentistry by any unregistered person. Those individuals who had not undertaken a formal qualification in dentistry could register with the Dental Board and they became known as 1921 dentists.

Unfortunately, the Act failed to formalise the position of dental dressers. The definition of 'minor dental work' undertaken in public services by persons other than registered dentists was not sufficiently detailed until September 1922. During that month, the Ministry of Health published the definition of minor dental work to exclude fillings and extractions. The work was limited to non-operative procedures. In addition, there were strict conditions of supervision, circulated to local authorities by the Board of Education. The dental dresser scheme was extended until the end of 1925 when the full implementation of the 1922 conditions would be strictly applied.

On January 24th 1925 Dr Barwise sadly died. He was undoubtedly the key driver for the development of dental dressers. Almost 100 years after his death, skill mix remains a difficult subject for the profession. There were attempts to retain the role of dental dresser. In 1926–27 the County Councils Association pressed the Board of Education on attempting to amend the 1921 Dentists Act to allow dental dressers to be employed. This was to no avail.

In 1930 the Hackney Wick Dental Clinic applied to the Ministry of Health to appoint dental dressers to treat those over school age and people who fell outside the remit of the school medical service. Two things were in their favour: the Minister was aware of the dental needs of schoolchildren and dental manpower resources were scarce. However, employment of dental dressers was still a sensitive area. Later in 1931 the Eastman Dental Clinic in London put forward a suggestion that the definition of minor dental work could be altered to allow nurses to undertake dental inspections in the School Medical

Service. The idea met with favour by Sir Francis Acland, chairman of the Dental Board. The dental profession was not supportive and opposed the idea and the Dental Board advised the Minister not to proceed. This closed the chapter on dental dressers or nurses with expanded duties for the time being. It is interesting to appreciate that the dental dresser was a dental nurse who was trained to undertake additional operational procedures and duties. It is erroneous to state that dental dressers were the forerunners of either dental hygiene or dental therapy.

Interestingly, during this period, civilian dental attendants were established as part of the demand for dental services by the Royal Navy, to ensure a permissible level of dental fitness for those in service. The early dental attendants were also supported by sick berth attendants – attendants who eventually were identified as sick berth attendants for dental services and who were not to undertake duties of the general sick berth attendant. They were identified as reservists, initially RSBA (D). Sick berthers for dentistry were identifiable by the distinct 'D' under the Red Cross sign on their badge. At one point, retired dental mechanics (technicians) were said to be acting as dental attendants. Dental surgeon students of the time also joined the Royal Navy Auxiliary Sick Berth Reserves. This all came to an end with postwar demobilisation. National service was introduced and eventually the Women's Royal Naval Service came about, with the first dental attendants qualifying in 1949 (Dawes and Holland 1995).

1940 saw the birth of the Dental Nurses and Assistants Society (DNAS) of Great Britain in Leyland, Lancashire. Dental nurses Amelia White and Madeleine (Bunty) Winter and dentist P.E. Grundy were the founders. Bunty was the Association's first General Secretary in the early 1940s. The Association today has a mission to: 'Empower dental nurses to advocate and advance the role of dental nursing through a platform of lifelong learning in order to enable a level of competently applied knowledge, skills and attitudes and behaviours related to the progression from novice to expert practice, that underpin the evolving demands of current and future oral healthcare for the UK population' (www.badn.org.uk).

In 1943 the Association held the first dental nurse examination and Bunty Winter was one of the first dental nurses to become qualified. The resulting British Dental Nurses and Assistants Examining Board

(BDNAEB) remained part of the Association until 1988, when it became a separate organisation. The name of the Board experienced another two iterations – the Examining Board for Dental Assistants (EBDA), then the National Examining Board for Dental Surgery Assistants (NEBDSA) before finally becoming the National Examining Board for Dental Nurses (NEBDN) in 1995. Only dentists were allowed to be examiners until 1978 when senior nurses were also accepted onto the Board. In 1989 postcertificate examinations were introduced. The Association set up a voluntary registration scheme for dental nurses/assistants in 1964 and became a trade union in the 1970s. From their first inception, with the exception of dental technology, the non-dentist dental professions have been the majority preserve of women.

Later in the 1940s, the British Society of Dental Assistants was established in London in 1943. However, this was dissolved in 1949 after failing to be recognised by the Whitley Council.

In 1948, the Confederation of Health Services Employees unsuccessfully attempted to recruit from DNAS members. Also in 1948, a British Dental Association-led inquiry looked into the conditions of work of dental assistants and proposed that 'an increased number of properly trained chairside assistants was desirable' (BDA 1948, p.10). The committee also stated that 'every normally busy practitioner should employ an assistant', but emphasised that the chairside assistant is an ancillary worker and 'that her work should be restricted to assisting the dentist without impinging upon the sphere of the dentist'.

Moving through the twentieth century, the concept of four-handed dentistry appeared in the late 1950s. Dalai et al. (2014) state that the term 'four-handed dentistry' was first recorded in the proceedings of a conference on 'training dental students to use chairside assistants' in 1960. Since then, this term has been widely used. Robinson et al. (1968) summarise the concept as follows: 'four-handed dentistry involves the co-ordinated work of both the dentist and assistant, working as a team to perform those operations in a manner that has been carefully and deliberately planned'. As well as being heralded as central to motion economy and contributing to reducing physical stresses, four-handed dentistry really celebrates the role of the dental nurse and the need to work differently and better, as a team. It is still celebrated and encouraged, and many now consider similar notions and concepts through the lens of human factors and ergonomics in dentistry (Ellwood 2022a).

In 1993 the Nuffield inquiry proved to be a turning point for modern dental nursing requirements. Ellwood (2022b) gives an excellent overview of the impact of Nuffield. In 1994–95 there was a change in the title of those assisting dentists from dental surgery assistant (DSA) back to dental nurse. At this time, dental nursing qualifications remained optional. The Dental Advisory Review Group (DARG) responded to the Nuffield report suggesting that all PCDs should be registered with the GDC if they were qualified or on an approved training course. By May 1999, the GDC agreed in principle to the suggestion and a steering group was formed in 2001 to implement this recommendation.

In the last quarter of the twentieth century, serious attention began to be paid to infection control and decontamination in dentistry. Interestingly, Nield (2020, p.15) tells us that 'all its (infection control) tenets were discovered or rediscovered in the nineteenth century and yet it took over a century for these findings to become everyday procedure'. Decontamination is a major area of responsibility for the dental nurse. Whilst all dental professionals in clinical practice are at risk from infectious hazards, in the primary care setting, it is the dental nurse who takes the lead in the handling of sharps and contaminated instruments. This role is crucial to the protection of patients and colleagues. See the twenty-first century section below for how health and safety regulations developed in this area. The list of infectious risks to those working in clinical dentistry is a long one, including viruses, bacterial, prions and fungi.

Figure 2.1 gives a stylised representation of progressive infection control challenges over time.

In 1993, the Department of Health issued guidance on hepatitis B vaccination. This required all staff primarily performing exposure-prone procedures to be immunised against hepatitis B and to have their serological response checked.

The first case of HIV/AIDS was reported in the UK in December 1981. Nield (2020, p.13) reported that 'the 1980s saw the emergence of HIV/AIDS and this along with the increasing prevalence of hepatitis B and C led to the introduction of sharps management procedures and the more widespread adoption of barrier protection and use of

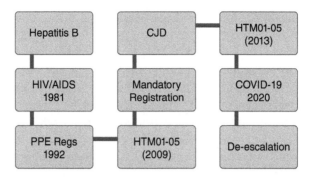

Figure 2.1 Infection control progression linked to major infections.

autoclaves, rather than boiling water for instrument sterilization'. Hot air ovens and glass beads should not be forgotten.

This heightened awareness of HIV/AIDS also saw patients needing reassurance and for a dental assistant working in that period, it was not uncommon to have to take patients into the decontamination room and demonstrate how the instruments were precleaned and sterilised. The research at the time showed that the transmission rate in dental settings was very low (McCarthy et al. 2002). However, it was this serious viral infection that triggered the routine use of gloves in dentistry. It is amazing to remember that there was considerable resistance to the wearing of gloves. There were reports of gloves being washed between patients and dental nurses often had to buy their own gloves. Unthinkable today (hopefully).

Personal protective equipment (PPE) regulations arrived in 1992, including the routine use of masks and spectacles in addition to gloves. Many dental nurses today are unlikely to recall a time when PPE was not provided. However, prior to the early 1990s PPE was not readily available and especially not for general use. At that time, some clinicians were charging team members for any PPE worn, something that may have been catastrophic given the COVID-19 pandemic which arrived in the UK in 2022.

A few years later in the late 1990s, cases of variant Creutzfeldt–Jakob disease (CJD) were diagnosed in humans and decontamination and infection control were in the spotlight again. The disease was caused by eating beef infected with the prion disease bovine spongiform encephalopathy (BSE) or 'mad cow' disease. Patients again became cautious about attending the dental surgery. Research demonstrated that CJD could be transmitted orally and was found in dental pulp. This led to the publication of the UK's first major guidelines on infection control in dentistry: 'Decontamination in primary care dental practices' (HTM 01-05) (DOH 2013). Published first in 2009 by the English Department of Health, modified in 2013, with minor amendments, it influenced later documents produced in the other UK countries. Scotland produced the Decontamination Into Practice document in 2007, which was updated in 2014. HTM 01-05 has become the overarching document which underpins guidelines in Wales, Scotland and Ireland. Other legislation exists in Northern Ireland (Regulation and Quality Improvement Authority 2013) and Scotland (SDCEP 2014). Whilst all follow a similar vein, there are subtle differences from region to region. Interestingly, Porter (2002) reported that there had never been any association between dental care and the transmission of CJD.

With the introduction of the Health Technical Memoranda (HTM) in 2009 and 2013, decontamination, infection prevention and control moved to a whole new level. This dramatic shift increased the workload for dental nurses, requiring training and a need to upskill. Dental nurses became involved in clinical audits, testing, recording and storage of data. Some were and continue to be involved in inspections and the training of new team members. Those dental nurses involved in education had to adapt their teaching and resources.

A major impact of the guidelines was the mandatory single-patient use of endodontic reamers and files to avoid prion transmission. There was also a greater emphasis on single-use instruments for other procedures and the washing and rinsing of instruments prior to sterilisation – not exactly a new requirement (Crabb 2013).

The focus on infection control and decontamination in dentistry shone a spotlight on accountability and responsibility, with dental nurses taking a leading role working within specified and ethical guidelines, essential to ensure the safety and well-being of patients and the whole team.

Role of the world wars

There can be little doubt that the two world wars had a considerable impact on the role of women and the work that they could undertake. Indirectly and directly, this will have impacted upon dental nursing.

Hall (2012) estimated that during the first world war (1914–1918) about two million women undertook jobs that had been previously undertaken by men before they went off to fight. During the Second World War, the number of women taking on traditionally male jobs is estimated at five million. Women got a taste for work outside the more traditional roles that had been deemed appropriate before the war(s). Society began to appreciate that women could successfully take on jobs that prior to the war would have been considered as impossible. Attitudes began to change both for individual women but also for the larger (male) population. The genie was well and truly out of the bottle.

Reed (2021) suggests that a primary factor in the emergence of training for dental nurses was the First World War. This resulted in a lack of men, which led local authorities and county medical officers to begin to employ and train dental nurses.

The Royal Air Force (RAF) Dental Branch was formed in 1930 as the importance of air power grew. By 1935 the RAF was served by 16 dental officers with permanent commissions, 29 with non-permanent/reserve commissions and 51 civilian practitioners. The RAF quickly recognised the need for 'dental clerk orderlies' to support dentists in the surgery and with administration. They were soon renamed as 'dental surgery attendants' and performed similar duties to a modern dental nurse (Webb 2021).

During World War II, trained and experienced dental nurses were recruited and employed by the armed forces. However, within general dental practices the employment of dental nurses was patchy, many dentists still choosing to work alone. There was no formal training for dental nurses so the best that could be hoped for was a dentist who was interested enough in education to train their dental nurse well.

Chapter 3 covers training and qualification and we see there that formal training began in the UK in 1943, during the Second World War. An interesting article by Loretz originally published in 1943 has been republished as part of the 'From the Archive' series in the British Dental Journal with commentary by Reed (2022). Loretz makes the case for trained dental nurses, and in particular she draws to the reader's attention the valuable contribution dental nurses make to safe dental care. Loretz is quite rightly concerned by the lack of understanding of asepsis and clean working conditions in the surgery. Reed (2022) further notes that this paper written towards the end of World War II 'brought dental nursing back to dentistry's collective conscious'.

Women in employment – twentieth and twenty-first centuries

This was the time when the previously largely unchallenged view of women's place as being within the home was blown apart.

The twentieth century saw a revolution in policies that supported women to work (Lewis et al. 2008). However, it is sobering to remember that many of these changes have only occurred in the last 30–40 years. From the late 1990s childcare provision was improved, but childcare in the UK was and is amongst the most expensive in Europe (Schober and Scott 2012). The Part-Time Work Directive (1997) gave part-time workers the same benefits as full-time workers. This included training, pay and parental leave, all of which would have an impact for dental nurses. Maternity leave became a statutory right in the 1999–2001 Employment Relations and Employment Act (Williams and Cohen-Cooper 2004). As important as the changes to the law supporting women in employment is society's attitude to women working outside the home. Attitudes and behaviours change over time and as more women work, it becomes the norm and acceptable. This opens the door to more women working until society views women working as expected.

The British Social Attitudes (BSA) survey, run by the National Centre for Social Research, has been carried out annually since 1983 (Park et al. 2013). Every year over 3000 people are asked what it's like to live in Britain. In the mid-1980s, the BSA survey reported that close to half (43% in 1984 and 48% in 1987) of the public supported a gendered separation of roles, with the man in the 'breadwinner' role and the woman in the 'caring' role. Clearly, at that time, there was a strong belief in the traditional gender divide. Since then, there has been a steady decline in the numbers of people who report holding this view. In 2022, only 13% of people – or one person in eight – think that this should be the case. So, in respect of whether women should stay at home rather than take on paid work, there has been a dramatic shift in attitudes to gender roles in the past 30–40 years in the UK. This decline is primarily a result of generational replacement, with consecutive generations being less supportive of traditional gender roles.

Furley (2015) notes that 'women today predominate in the "caring" occupations such as medical nursing, carers and nursery education.' Why is this? Is it the natural order of things that women are more compassionate, more empathic, more caring? Or is it a lingering of the old order of things that until relatively recently saw men configuring the world and having more power and control? Perhaps this notion of women as carers is not as accurate as it at first appears. As noted earlier in the chapter, Barrett-Landau and Henle (2014) suggest that nursing has been portrayed only as a feminine occupation since the appearance of the Nightingale nursing training style in the mid nineteenth century which favoured women over men to become nurses. Prior to that, nursing was a male occupation. As some of the art record demonstrates, male assistants assisted male dentists for much of the time.

Irvine et al. (2022) noted that in September 2021 in the UK, the most common sectors in which to find working women were health and social work, accounting for 21% of all jobs held by women. Within the sector, women predominated, with 78% of jobs held by women. These data are sourced from the Office for National Statistics (ONS) workforce jobs series, and are a count of jobs rather than people as one person may hold multiple jobs.

In 2021, 24% of women worked in professional occupations, compared to around 23% of men, but women were more likely than men to work part-time.

The employment rate for UK women was 72.1% in July–September 2021 which compared to 63.7% in the European Union, 65.1% in North America and 71.5% in Japan. The highest rate of female employment over this period could be found in Iceland (79%) (OECD 2021).

The ONS (2013) describes how the persistence of gendered job roles leaves females at a relative disadvantage in the labour market. Within dentistry, dental nurses receive the lowest pay of all the categories of dental professionals.

Finally, and pertinently with regard to gender in dental nursing, Furley (2015) makes a very good observation about dental nurses in the UK.

'Dental nursing remains relatively low paid and insecure, with many nurses being employed on the now notorious 'zero-hour contracts'. The upshot is that women find themselves undertaking work that men would traditionally not be willing to do, largely due to the pay and conditions associated with it. In addition, anecdotally, there appears to be reluctance on the behalf of dentists to employ male nurses as there is an expectation from the patient that nurses will be women.'

All of Furley's points make for interesting consideration. The question must be asked whether there is also a reluctance on the part of the profession itself that perhaps considers male dental nurses not wholly acceptable.

In 2022 dental nursing in the UK has a gender breakdown of about 86% women and 14% men employed within the profession (GDC 2022).

The twenty-first century

Important changes in decontamination straddled the end of the twentieth century and the beginning of the twenty-first century. In secondary dental care settings, central sterile services departments (CSSD) became commonplace. These departments clean, disinfect and sterilise reusable medical equipment, including dental equipment and instruments.

Early in the century, the move towards statutory registration for dental nurses began to quicken. In 2003, in response to the Nuffield Report, the Dental Auxiliaries (Amendment) Regulations 2003-11-07 Section 60 of the Health Act 1999 (column 1.047) makes clear that the plans for the historic shift to include dental nurses as registrants were progressing.

The Dentists Act 1984 (Amendment) Order 2005 introduced compulsory indemnity cover and allowed the GDC to regulate the whole dental team, including dental nurses and dental technicians, and to take action in cases of poor professional performance.

In 2006, a two-year window opened for registration. It offered three routes to allow existing dental nurses entry to the register by:
- qualification
- demonstrating competence via successful completion of the Access to Registration Training (ART), and

- the grandparenting route, which required supporting references and a need to have worked as a dental nurse for a minimum of four years in any eight-year period.

By 2006, the umbrella term of PCD had become dental care professionals (DCP), which is commonly applied today. The term, whilst covering all dental professionals including dentists, is generally taken to mean all dental care professionals except dentists.

In 2008, the time-limited grandparenting route and competence-based training period were brought to an end. Also at this time, statutory registration became compulsory via qualification only. Those with qualifications obtained before 1994 needed to have joined the register before the 2008 window closed to avoid having to retake their qualification. There was considerable confusion at the time and some missed the registration window.

2008 was a momentous year for dental nursing, dental nurses and indeed the whole dental profession. This was the year the profession of dental nursing was finally truly born, when dental nurses became registrants and were required to register with the GDC. It was a major milestone in the history of UK dental nursing and confirmed that dental nursing was a profession. Following mandatory registration, expanded duties training took hold and dental nurses began to establish themselves as valued members of the dental family. Continual professional development (CPD) and indemnity requirements came hand in hand with statutory registration. There will be more discussion of these topics in Chapter 3. Accountability, responsibility and working within specified and ethical guidelines came to the fore for individual dental nurses and such ways of working continue to be essential to the safety and well-being of patients and the team.

Another key moment in UK dental nursing history was the introduction of allowable clinical activity. The application of fluoride varnish by dental nurses was deemed appropriate either under prescription of a dentist or as part of a public health programme under the guidance of a dental public health consultant. The first programme in England was funded in 2008 and overseen by Dr Colette Bridgman. This was closely followed by Scotland on the back of the action plan for modernising the dental services in Scotland, known as the Childsmile programme (Macpherson et al. 2010), and then by Wales in 2009 (Iomhair et al. 2020). The programme in Wales is known as Design to Smile. This body of work was seen as a positive step along with tooth-brushing programmes to help improve the oral health of children.

At about this time, the profession decided not to use the title of registered dental nurse (RDN), as it was felt to not reflect the registrable title. It could also have been confused with the North American title of registered dental assistant.

With mandatory registration came the requirement for dental nurses to be indemnified, as all registered dental professionals must be. Each year dental nurses applying for initial or renewed registration or those applying for restoration need to make a declaration that they have indemnity cover in place or will have by the time they start practising.

Dental nurses may be covered by their employer's indemnity policy but they must have access to the policy and the GDC is at pains to point out that the responsibility lies with the dental nurse to ensure that they are appropriately covered. This not only applies to additional duties, but in some cases employer's policies offer no assistance in relation to regulatory hearings and matters of professional conduct. This applies in the case of both primary and secondary care and also within the corporate world as well as the military and community settings. It is a wise dental nurse who closely checks the indemnity cover they have. If you are a registered dental nurse regardless of whether you work clinically or non-clinically, indemnity is a mandatory requirement of registration.

In 2013, the Health & Safety (Sharp Instruments in Healthcare) Regulations made it clear that, with regard to sharps, the operator must take responsibility for correct use and disposal. Where dental nurses have a role in the handling of sharps, they must be trained accordingly.

The GDC Scope of Practice (2013) outlines the skills that dental nurses are required to demonstrate and lists the dental activities which can be carried out on prescription from a dentist or under the direction of another registrant. It also makes it clear that dental nurses do not diagnose disease or treatment plan. They are, however, allowed to undertake fluoride varnish application, not only under prescription from a dentist but as part of a structured dental health programme.

In just over 100 years, the role of the dental nurse has gone two steps forward (dental dressers) and one step back. Having said that, the opportunities for career and personal development are now very much wider and deeper than for dental nurses at the beginning of the twentieth century. More of that in Chapter 5. We shall have to see what the future holds.

This century has seen the dental nursing agency landscape grow beyond recognition. There are more self-employed dental nurses than ever before and this is perhaps the start of a reconfiguration of the workforce. In some instances, dental nurses are working in the dental trade industry, although when reviewing the census data, this is perhaps not a new move as women were reporting working in the trade industry during the twentieth entury. Dental nurses are also to be found in research and higher education institutions.

The world of social enterprise has found a place in dentistry. Where once the dental environment was predominantly NHS with a small amount of private work being undertaken, we are seeing a distinct shift. Corporate dentistry is another expansion area that has brought a very different dimension to working within dentistry.

In 2015 the Society of British Dental Nurses (SBDN) was founded by a number of experienced dental nurses. It had a key focus on the development of dental nurses through education, learning and training. The SBDN's mission is to inspire and engage dental nurses at every stage of their career, and a shift in thinking can be seen as they emphasise 'the here and now, and the future landscape of dentistry' (www.sbdn.org.uk). The society has evolved and expanded its work and added to its expert consultant board, its regional representatives and the ambassador team from across all the UK nations.

In 2018 the first ever faculty for dental care professionals was launched in Wales with the support of the then Chief Dental Officer, Dr Colette Bridgman. The faculty is known as the All Wales Faculty for Dental Care Professionals and is part of Bangor University. Two of the key members driving the work forward were integral to dental nursing, both holding dental nursing registration status with the GDC (https://awfdcp.ac.uk/).

The impact of viral infections again reared its head, as the COVID-19 pandemic had a huge impact on every aspect of our personal and professional lives. March 2020 saw a seismic shift and decontamination and infection prevention again took centre stage in healthcare. Dentistry was particularly affected in the early days of the pandemic. The response by all dental professionals required adaptability and flexibility. When it came to fallow time and managing the cleaning of surgeries, dental nurses were at the forefront of it all. Donning and doffing PPE became second nature. Those who were part of the think tank producing recommendations from research at speed found it to be a truly mind-blowing experience and a privilege. New and revised standard operating procedures came thick and fast from all four UK nations. There were variations, but with the same intended outcomes and a central helpline was so important for the dental nurses trying to manage the changes. Canada and North America both reported similar patterns and challenges even though as countries we were at different stages.

Many dental nurses were furloughed during the pandemic, some worked in urgent care settings and many secondary care and community service dental nurses were redeployed.

A number of dental professionals stepped outside dentistry at this time and took on roles in general medicine to support hospitals as they dealt with the unprecedented numbers of patients in intensive care. Dental nurses supported their general nurse colleagues in prone wards, turning severely ill patients. Dental nurses who ran the Rochdale care home became integral to their care of vulnerable older patients. Some teams in Scotland became involved in the vaccination schemes. At that time of global crisis, dental nurses stepped up to the plate and demonstrated their commitment, quick thinking, flexibility and adaptability to wider healthcare.

The pandemic certainly brought challenges at all levels. Dental nurses have been key in the management and maintenance of infection prevention and control. Sadly, as a direct result of the pandemic many dental nurses lost their employment and others simply decided to leave the profession.

2021 saw the launch of the DSA Alumni in the UK, which marked the sad loss of Dame Margaret Seward, an influential figure during times of enormous change for the then DSAs.

National Dental Nurses Day in the UK was launched in 2016 and is celebrated on 22nd November annually. This date recognises the first dental nursing examination held in 1943 in the UK.

The International Federation of Dental Assistants and Nurses (https://IFDAN.org) was founded in 2022. This exciting and ground-breaking federation brings together the Canadian Dental Assistants Association, the American Dental Assistants Association and the Society of British Dental Nurses. Representatives from these three organisations have been collaborating to establish the first international federation representing dental assistants and dental nurses from around the world. The three founding partners are looking to formally link national dental assisting/dental nursing professional associations from around the globe in a not-for-profit professional federation.

The overarching goal of the international group is to foster leadership and collaboration while acting as the principal advocate and promoter of the dental assisting/dental nursing profession globally. While improving and advancing the profession, the group will also promote global excellence in practice, research and education and will advocate for improved oral health measures/initiatives worldwide.

In this chapter, we have seen dental nursing evolve and grow to become a vital profession within the family of dentistry. Dental nursing can rightly be seen as a career and not merely a job (a paid position of regular employment). The dictionary definition of a career (noun) is: 'an occupation or profession, especially one requiring special training, followed as one's lifework' (www. dictionary.com). There can be no question that dental nursing has developed from a surgery chaperone, a 'lady in waiting', to a vital and valuable member of the team providing care and treatment for patients.

There is so much to be proud of in the emergence of dental nursing as a profession and the hard work of dental nurses both in the UK and across the globe. Yes, there have been low points, as is only to be expected, but dental nurses can hold their heads high.

In the next chapter, we take a more global perspective on dental nursing and consider how the profession of dental nursing developed outside the United Kingdom.

Note

Census data have been taken from the 'Find my past' website: www. findmypast.co.uk. This is a subscription genealogical database. Records of UK census returns from 1841 to 1921 can be searched on line.

Pocket dentistry (https://pocketdentistry.com) is a search engine for clinical dental questions.

References

Acland, F. (1919). *Report of the Committee Appointed by the Lord President of Privy Council to Enquire into the Extent and Gravity of the Evils of Dental Practice by Persons Not Qualified under The Dentists Act, 1878*. HMSO, London, p.37.

Barrett-Landau, S., Henle, S. (2014). Men in nursing: their influence in a female dominated career. *Journal of Leadership Instruction*, **13**(2), 10–13.

Barwise, S. (1910). Treatment of school children. *Journal of the Royal Society for the Promotion of Health*, **31**, issue 3. Available at: https://ur.bookssc.me

Barwise, S. (1924). Dental dressers. *Lancet*, **204**(5276), 781–782.

Benazzi, S., Kullmer, O., Schulz, D., Gruppioni, G., Weber, G.W. (2013). Individual tooth macrowear pattern guides the reconstruction of Sts 52 (*Australopithecus africanus*) dental arches. *American Journal of Biological Anthropology*, **150**, 324–329.

British Dental Association, Incorporated Dental Society, Public Dental Service Association (1948). *Committee of Enquiry into the Training, Wages, Conditions of Service and Title of Women Assisting Dentists in Public or Private Service*. British Dental Association, London, p.10.

Brooks, J.A. (2019). *100 Years of Women in the Dental Profession in the UK, 1918–2018*. Cambridge University Press/Cambridge Scholars Publishing, Cambridge

Bullough, V.L. (1994). Men, women and nursing history. *Journal of Professional Nursing*, **10**(3), 127.

Crabb, C. (2013). How to create a sterile field: the dental nurses' role. *Dental Nursing*, **8**(4).

Dalai, D.R., Bhaskar, D.J., Agali, C.R., Gupta, V., Singh, N., Bumb, S.S. (2014). Four handed dentistry: an indispensable part for efficient clinical practice. *International Journal of Advances in Health Science*, **1**(1), 16–20.

Dawes, N.G., Holland, J.V. (1995). *A History of Dentistry in the Royal Navy 1905–1964*. Royal Society of Medicine Press, London.

Dentists Act 1984 (Amendment) Order 2005. Available at: www.legislation.gov.uk/uksi/2005/2011/made

Department of Health (DOH) (1993). *Protecting Healthcare Workers and Patients from Hepatitis B. Recommendations of the Advisory Group on Hepatitis*. HMSO, London.

Department of Health (DOH) (2013). *Decontamination in Primary Care Dental Practices*. HTM 01-05. Department of Health, London. Available at: www.england.nhs.uk/wp-content/uploads/2021/05/HTM_01-05_2013.pdf

Dussault, G. (1981). The professionalisation of dentistry. A study of occupational strategies (1900–1957). PhD thesis submitted to the University of London.

Ellwood, F. (2022a). The blame game has no place in dentistry (PowerPoint presentation). Available at: www.sbdn.org.uk

Ellwood, F. (2022b). The history of dental nursing. a 25 year perspective. Availableat:https://dentistry.co.uk/2022/06/01/the-history-of-dental-nursing-a-25-year-perspective/

Forshaw, R.J. (2009a). Dental health and disease in ancient Egypt. *British Dental Journal*, **206**, 421–424.

Forshaw, R.J. (2009b). The practice of dentistry in ancient Egypt. *British Dental Journal*, **206**(9), 481–486.

Forshaw, R.J. (2013). Hesyre: the first recorded physician and dental surgeon in history. *Bulletin of the John Rylands Library*, **1**, 181–202.

Furley, J. (2015). Equality in 2015: can dentistry hold its head high? Available at:www.gdpuk.com/blogs/entry/1300-equality-in-2015-can-dentistry-hold-its-head-high

Fuss, J., Uhlig, G., Bohme, M. (2018). Earliest evidence of caries lesion in hominids reveal sugar-rich diet for a Middle Miocene dryopithecine from Europe. *PLoS One*, **13**(8), e0203307.

Gelbier, S. (2005). 125 years of developments in dentistry, 1880–2005 Part 5: Dental education, training and qualifications. *British Dental Journal*, **199**, 685–688.

General Dental Council (2013). Scope of Practice. Available at: www.gdc-uk.org

General Dental Council (2022). Registration report. Available at: www.gdc-uk.org

Hall, L.A. (2012). *Sex, Gender and Social Change in Britain since 1890*, 2nd edn. Palgrave Macmillan, Basingstoke.

Harrison, T. (2021). Florence Nightingale's legacy on the role of men in community nursing. *British Journal of Community Nursing*, **26**(6), 302–306.

Health and Safety (Sharp Instruments In Healthcare) Regulations (2013). Available at: www.hse.gov.uk/pubns/hsis7.htm

Irvine, S., Clark, H., Ward, M., Francis-Devine, B. (2022). Women and the UK economy. Research Briefing. House of Commons Library, No. 6838. Available at: https://researchbriefings.files.parliament.uk/documents/SN06838/SN06838.pdf

Iomhair, A.N., Wilson, M., Morgan, M. (2020) Ten years of Designed to Smile in Wales. *BDJ Team*, **7**, 12–15. Available at: www.nature.com/articles/s41407-020-0285-1

Lewis, J., Campbell, M., Huerta, C. (2008). Patterns of paid and unpaid work in Western Europe. *Journal of European Social Policy*, **18**(1), 21–37.

Loretz, M.M. (1943). The importance of surgery assistance and maintenance: a plea for the employment of the trained dental nurse. *British Dental Journal*, **75**, 34–38.

Macpherson, L.M.D., Ball, G.E., Brewster, L., et al. (2010). Childsmile: the national child oral health improvement programme in Scotland. Part 1: establishment and development. *British Dental Journal*, **209**, 73–78.

McCarthy, G.M., Sali, C.S., Bednarsh, H., Wangrangsimalaul, K., Jorge, J., Page-Shafer, K. (2002). Transmission of HIV in the dental clinic and elsewhere. *Oral Disease*, **8**(suppl 2), 126–135.

Mortimer, I. (2009). *The Time Traveller's Guide to Medieval England*. Vintage Books, London.

Nield, H. (2020). A short history of infection control in dentistry. *BJD Team*, **7**(8), 12–15. Available at: www.nature.com/articles/s41407-020-0402-1

Office for Economic Co-operation and Development (OECD) (2021). Labour force short-term statistics. Available at: https://stats.oecd.org/index.aspx?queryid=35253

Office for National Statistics (ONS) (2013). Full report: Women in the labour market. Available at: www.ons.gov.uk/employmentandlabourmarket/peopleinwork/employmentandemployeetypes/articles/womeninthelabourmarket/2013-09-25#:~:text=In%20April%20to%20June%202013%2C%20looking%20at%20the%20not%20seasonally,average%20hours%20worked%20per%20week.

Park, A., Bryson, C., Clery, E., Curtice, J., Phillips, M. (eds) (2013). British Social Attitudes: 30th Report. Available at: www.basw.co.uk/system/files/resources/basw_22805-8_0.pdf

Platt, A. (trans.) (2015). Aristotle. On the Generation of Animals, Book IV, part 6. Available at: www.esp.org/books/aristotle/generation-of-animals/#:~:text=The%20Generation%20of%20Animals%20(or,early%20days%20of%20classical%20genetics.

Porter, S.R. (2002). Prions and dentistry. *Journal of the Royal Society of Medicine*, **95**(4), 178–181.

Purvis, J. (1991). *A History of Women's Education in England*. McGraw-Hill Education/Open University Press, Buckingham.

Raitapuro-Murray, T., Molleson, T.I., Hughes, F.J. (2014). The prevalence of periodontal disease in a Romano-British population c. 200–400 AD. *British Dental Journal*, 217, 459–466.

Reed, D. (2021). The history of dental nursing. *BDJ Team*, **8**, 48–51.

Reed, D. (2022). Expert commentary. *British Dental Journal*, **233**, 213–214.

Regulation and Quality Improvement Authority, Northern Ireland. (2013). Updated Northern Ireland guidance on decontamination in primary care dental practices. Available at: https://hscbusiness.hscni.net/pdf/PEL%2013-13%20UPDATED%20NI%20GUIDANCE.pdf

Ridley, S. (2017). *Suffragettes and the Fight for the Vote*. Watts Publishing Group, London.

Robinson, G.E., Wuehrmann, A. H., Sinnett, G.M., McDevitt, E.J. (1968). Four handed dentistry: the whys and wherefores. *Journal of the American Dental Association*, **77**(3), 573–579.

Ross, D. (2017). Challenges for men in a female dominated environment. *Links to Health and Social Care*, 2(1), 4–20.

Schober, P., Scott, J. (2012). Maternal employment and gender role attitudes: dissonance among British men and women in the transition to parenthood. *Work, Employment and Society*, **26**(3), 514–530.

Scottish Dental Clinical Effectiveness Programme (SDCEP) (2014). *Decontamination in Practice: Dental Clinical Guidelines*. Available at: www.sdcep.org.uk

Symes, R.A. (1995). Educating women: the preceptress and her pen. PhD thesis, University of York, Centre for Women's Studies.

Takayanagi, M. (2018). 'One of the most revolutionary proposals that has ever been put before the House': the passage of the Parliament (Qualification of Women) Act 1918. In: Black, L., Carr, R. (eds) *Labour, British Radicalism and the First World War*. Manchester University Press, Manchester, pp.56–72.

Tomes, C.S. (1919) Report of the Dentists' Act Committee. *British Dental Journal*, **40**(5), 177–178.

Vallano, A. (2008) *Your Career in Nursing: Manage Your Future in the Challenging World of Health Care*. Kaplan Publishing, New York.

Webb, C. (2021). The History of Dentistry: Dentistry in the RAF. Available at: https://pearldentalsoftware.com/marketing-team/dental-history-raf-dental-branch/

Williams, J.C., Cohen-Cooper, H. (2004). The public policy of motherhood. *Journal of Social Issues*, **60**(4), 849–865.

Chapter 3   **The rise of the profession**

Having considered the early history of dental nursing and particularly the establishment of dental nursing within the UK, this chapter will take a wider view of dental nursing outside the UK. We will include New Zealand, Canada and North America but also Europe and touch lightly on other countries across the world. Comparisons will be made to show the difference in content of roles across the globe and consider the wider social and gender perspectives. The chapter will trace the profession of dental nursing and how a job became the profession it is today. We will look at the ups and downs, the pros and cons for dental nurses and dentistry as the profession is developed and launched. The ramifications and impact on individuals and the working environment are also reviewed.

The primary role of the dental assistant has been identified historically by many as assisting the dentist. What is clear is that not every dentist worked with a dental assistant and their education and training appear to have been poles apart. This could simply be because not all countries recognise being a dental assistant as a professional role. In many countries there is minimal regulation around dental activity, and few countries articulate that the dental assistant must undertake formal training. Even fewer insist on dental assistants being formally registered with a dental regulator.

The evolution of the profession of dentistry and those who worked within it took place across the world and was not confined to the UK. Development of the field has varied considerably over the years and the differences appear to have been influenced by a wide range of factors. These have included times of war, increase in disease burden, workforce shortages, population increase, legislation, regulation, hierarchy, professionalisation, professional protectionism, financial

How to Develop Your Career in Dental Nursing, First Edition. Edited by Janine Brooks and Fiona Ellwood.
© 2023 John Wiley & Sons Ltd. Published 2023 by John Wiley & Sons Ltd.

constraints, economic disruption and most recently the COVID-19 pandemic. In modern-day Britain, contractual arrangements have also been identified as influencing the dental nursing field.

Over the years, the role and responsibilities of the dental nurse have evolved. As discussed in some detail in the previous chapter, when considering this evolution, it is important to consider the various terms and compilations that have been applied to the role over the years. Of equal interest are the commonalities of these across nations and countries, as well as their disparateness. Most commonly and synonymously applied historically and in modernity is the term 'dental assistant' but it is interesting that the UK moved away from this title as professional registration came to the fore.

When considering the identity of the modern-day dental nurse in the UK, it must be acknowledged that when comparing and contrasting to the role of the dental assistant, they are unequivocally alike, if not identical. This is not the case worldwide. In North America alone, up to 40 different job titles were found as part of research conducted in 2015 (OHWRC 2015). The most frequently applied are given below.

Subordinate	Dental house maiden	Auxiliary
	Dental nurse	
Lady in waiting	Chairside attendants	Certified dental assistant
Licensed dental assistant	Dental assistant	Dental auxiliaries
Stomatological assistant	Chairside assistant	Registered dental assistant
Trained auxiliary		

Considering the wider global landscape of dental nursing, we find dental nurses and dental assistants begin to appear from the last quarter of the nineteenth century and the early twentieth century. Dental assistants were first reported in North America, albeit as 'ladies in waiting' in 1885. Reed (2021) notes that in Berlin, dental nurses assisted dentists from 1909. New Zealand and North America first alluded to dental assistants in 1917, followed closely by Canada in 1919. In England, although there is mention of dental assistants in 1909 as someone assisting the dentist, there appears to be little written relating to dental assistants in the UK until the 1940s. However, as noted in Chapter 2, the 1881 census for England shows one dental nurse, called Fanny Payne, a single 35 year old who lived in St Martin in the Fields, London, and worked as a nurse at the dental hospital, probably the Royal Dental Hospital which opened in 1858. This record predates North America by four years. Presumably there were other dental nurses working, although none are recorded in the 1871 UK census.

It is not possible to give detailed information for every country in relation to dental nursing/dental assistants, but we have included a little for Europe and the wider world. Our central focus for dental assistants outside the UK is North America, Canada and New Zealand. Representatives from the Canadian Dental Assistants Association, the American Dental Assistants Association and the Society of British Dental Nurses have established the first international federation representing dental assistants and dental nurses – the International Federation for Dental Assistants and Dental Nurses (IFDAN). Colleagues from Canada and North America have kindly assisted us with information from their countries.

North America

The first verifiable report of a dentist working with an assistant in North America is found in 1885. The wife of Dr Edmund Kells, a New Orleans dentist, began to assist her husband in his surgery. She was not given the title of dental nurse or even dental assistant, she was a 'lady in attendance'. This title gives the impression that Mrs Kells could have simply been present in the surgery whilst her husband operated and tended to his patients. It is likely her duties would have been quite menial, perhaps mostly cleaning up after surgery and chaperoning female patients. Whatever she did seems to have been a success because as the practice grew, Dr Kells took on another lady in attendance, Malvina Cueria. Malvina is reported to be the first dental assistant in modern history and she was only a teenager when she began her career. She and no doubt others like her within the surgery made it possible for women to have dental treatment undertaken without needing to be accompanied by their husbands or other male relative.

Malvina Cueria went on to serve as an American Dental Assistants Association district trustee from 1953 to 1956. At the age of 87, she was honoured by that professional organisation and spoke of her experiences as a dental assistant at a convention in New Orleans in 1980. Malvina died on December 4, 1991 at the age of 98.

Another pioneer dental assistant was Juliette A. Southard. She was employed by New York City dentist Dr Henry Fowler, in the early 1900s. Juliette formed a local dental assistants society in 1921 in New York, following the first North American dental assistants society which formed in Nebraska in 1917. The American Dental Assistants Association (ADAA) was founded in 1924 by Juliette and it is the oldest and largest association dedicated to making dental assisting a profession. The ADAA has about 20 000 members (2022).

North America has a system of building credentials and working toward the Dental Assisting National Board certification. Rather than advancing general skills, dental assistants in North America can complete certification in six core specialist fields.

- Anatomy, morphology, physiology, infection prevention and radiation health and safety training
- General chairside radiation safety and infection prevention and component exams
- Orthodontic assisting and infection prevention
- Coronal polishing, sealants and topical fluoride
- Impressions, temporaries, sealants and restorative functions
- Infection prevention and control

In those unregulated provinces and states, additional duties are deemed as being permissible, reversible and delegable duties. The roles and levels of confusion about the various roles appear to bemuse many. With additional workloads come additional titles.

Each additional qualification is represented as being 'certified' in the chosen field, for example Certificate in Dental Infection Prevention and Control (CDIPC). The dental assistant will be identified as having expanded functions – expanded function dental assistant or EFDA. In the unregulated states, unregulated dental assistants might undertake these duties without certification and can be trained on the job. Dental assistants can expect to earn more with certificated duties.

Currently, the potential number of dental assistants in North America is approximately 350 317, with 12% being certified; it is not mandatory to be certified to work. Ninety-five percent of North American dental nurses are female and the average age is 35 years. The vast majority of dental nurses in North America work in private practice.

A recent development in Texas is strict guidance on the ethical practice of applying teledentistry as part of the dental assistant's workload. North America has also been ahead of the game when it comes to the purposeful application of fluoride varnish and the ability to apply silver diamine fluoride. I am sure many of you will be asking when this will come to the UK (ADAA 2022).

New Zealand

In some ways, the evolution of the New Zealand school dental nurse mirrors the country's distinctive geography and demography. The country has two main large islands and a relatively sparse population outside the cities and towns. In 1950, the population of New Zealand was 1.8 million, with a high proportion of young people. Wellington, Auckland, Christchurch and Dunedin, the biggest cities, were not particularly large by European standards. The largest had a maximum population of 300 000. The bulk of the population lived in small townships of 2–3000 people, and in rural communities. In March 2022, the population had risen to over 5 million.

In 1921, New Zealand opened the first training school for dental nurses, situated in Wellington (Moffat et al. 2017). In April of that year, 30 women aged between 18 and 36 years began training as dental nurses for the state-funded School Dental Service (SDS). The first school dental nurses graduated in April 1923. The SDS was established to provide New Zealand primary schoolchildren with free dental care, in recognition of the appalling condition of their teeth – nine out of ten were said to be in need of dental treatment. The social policy of the time was also heavily focused on children's health and well-being.

The school dental nurses undertook much of the responsibility for the dental health of schoolchildren. They carried out examinations, cavity preparation, restorations, pulp capping and extraction of deciduous teeth.

The New Zealand model was replicated in Australia, remote parts of Canada and in The Netherlands. The New Zealand school dental nurse was an important influence on the emergence of systems of oral healthcare, particularly in South East Asia, where a number of countries also adopted the New Zealand model.

The model was not without its detractors and the upskilling of women to provide dental care in schools was opposed by the medical and trained nurses' associations, which held protest meetings around the country and made submissions to the government. These groups argued that training dental nurses would be less cost- and time-effective than employing already trained male dentists, and some feared it would lower professional standards. The training school continued in operation until 1999. Fifteen other countries set up similar schemes.

Canada

In 1926 Marion Edwards began to organise dental assistants in eastern Canada and the Canadian Dental Assistants Association was formed. Registration or licensure of dental assistants in Canada rests with the provincial dental assisting regulatory associations (DARA), often referred to as a 'regulatory college'.

In 1960, the higher standards for national certification were established and in 1968 the first 136 members successfully completed the national certificate. In 1997 the National Dental Assisting Examining Board (NDAEB) was formed to oversee the national certification and examination process. Interestingly, the first international dental assisting and dental nursing symposium was held in conjunction with the ADAA.

Of further interest was the introduction of a jointly funded research grant venture in 2014 (James 2016) and as a result of this the first research paper, entitled 'Building capacity in dental assisting research: the self-reported impact of occupational health stressors on the work-life of Canadian dental assistants', was published in 2016. It becomes apparent from this paper that there was an overwhelming outcry to have pan-Canadian structure and co-ordination regarding regulation, education and skills for all dental assistants. Thomson (2015) alludes to a number of reports prior to 2014 that made recommendations for dental assisting to be recognised as a profession in Quebec (Hall Report 1964, Wells Report 1970, Bernier Report 2012), but all recommendations so far have been both delayed and adamantly opposed by organised dentistry.

Dental assistants in some provinces in Canada are classified as either level I (chairside assistant) or level II (trained in intraoral duties). A level I dental assistant works closely with and under the supervision of a dentist, performing tasks before and after the dentist meets the patient and assists during procedures. Moving to level II allows the dental assistant to effectively undertake level II clinical tasks. They are identified as multi-skilled professionals and self-sufficient practitioners providing direct patient care and support procedures, through delegation of duties sanctioned by legislation. These are outlined in Table 3.1 where duties in Canada, North America and the UK are compared and contrasted.

In 2022 there are 26 000–29 000 dental assistants working in Canada, with almost 20 000 registered with a provincial dental assisting association. Of those 20 000, approximately 74% are certified or licensed, neither of which is mandatory. Ninety-nine percent of Canadian dental nurses are female and the highest concentration of average age is 19–25 year olds and the lowest is the 46–50 year old group (CDAA 2022).

United Kingdom

In September 2022 in the UK, there were 57 993 registered dental nurses: 57 158 female and 835 male (1.4%) (GDC 2022). Prior to registration, a UK dental nurse needs to have successfully completed an approved qualification in dental nursing. As with all categories of dental professional in the UK, the title of dental nurse is legally protected and only those qualified and registered with the GDC may use the title. It should be noted that dental + nurse must be used together for the legal protection to be applied, as the title 'nurse' is legally protected and applied to general nurses. Education providers need to be approved by the GDC and undergo regular reviews. There is currently no means of knowing how many student/trainee dental nurses there are in the UK. The acronym RDN (registered dental nurse) is not a registrable title acknowledged by the GDC nor is extended duties dental nurse (EDDN).

Dental nurses in the UK have a clearly defined scope of practice and all registrants must work within their scope of practice. There is a list of possible additional duties which can only be undertaken after referral and prescription from the dentist or other appropriate registrant. All dental nurses must be confident, competent, registered, indemnified

Table 3.1 Basic dental nurse duties comparison – North America, Canada and the UK.

North America	Canada	United Kingdom
The dental assistant is recognised as assisting the dentist and dental hygienist during a variety of treatment procedures; their duties may vary across states	Throughout Canada dental assisting is identified as a 'restricted healthcare occupation'. Basic duties may be province specific	Dental nurses are identified as registered dental professionals, who provide clinical support to registrants and patients
Taking and developing dental radiographs (x-rays)	Taking and developing dental radiographs (x-rays)	Prepare equipment, materials and patients for radiography and process radiographs. Do **NOT** take radiographs – post basic qualification required
Asking about the patient's medical history and taking blood pressure and pulse	Asking about the patient's medical history and taking blood pressure and pulse	Taking blood pressure and pulse not part of duties
Serving as an infection control officer, developing infection control protocol, and preparing and sterilising instruments and equipment	Serving as an infection control officer, developing infection control protocol, and preparing and sterilising instruments and equipment	Carry out infection prevention and control to prevent contamination
Helping patients feel comfortable before, during and after dental treatment	Helping patients feel comfortable before, during and after dental treatment	Monitor, support and reassure patients
Providing patients with instructions for oral care following surgery or other dental procedures, such as the placement of a restoration	Providing patients with instructions for oral care following surgery or other dental procedures, such as the placement of a restoration	Give appropriate patient advice

(Continued)

Table 3.1 (Continued)

North America	Canada	United Kingdom
Teaching patients appropriate oral hygiene strategies to maintain oral health (e.g. tooth brushing, flossing and nutritional counselling)	Teaching patients appropriate oral hygiene strategies to maintain oral health (e.g. tooth brushing, flossing and nutritional counselling)	Post basic qualification generally required
Taking impressions of patients' teeth for study casts (models of teeth)	Taking impressions of patients' teeth for study casts (models of teeth)	Post basic qualification required
Performing office management tasks that often require the use of a computer	Performing office management tasks that often require the use of a computer	Similar duties
Communicating with patients and suppliers (e.g. scheduling appointments, answering the telephone, billing and ordering supplies)	Communicating with patients and suppliers (e.g. scheduling appointments, answering the telephone, billing and ordering supplies)	Similar duties, although dental receptionist may undertake these duties
Helping to provide direct patient care in all dental specialties, including orthodontics, paediatric dentistry, periodontics and oral surgery	Assisting with and helping to provide direct patient care in all dental specialties, including orthodontics, paediatric dentistry, periodontics and oral surgery	Prepare and maintain the clinical environment Record dental charting and oral tissue assessment carried out by clinicians Prepare mix and handle biomaterials Keep accurate and contemporaneous patient records Support patients and colleagues if there is a medical emergency Make appropriate referrals to other health professionals

Table 3.1 (Continued)

North America	Canada	United Kingdom
Treatment procedures, such as the placement of a restoration (filling)	Treatment procedures, such as the placement of a restoration (filling)	Post basic qualification required for limited treatment procedures

and trained to undertake additional skills. Occasionally dental nurses with additional skills are referred to as having extended duties.

Table 3.1 helps to identify the similarities and differences within the UK, Canada and North America. What is obvious is that both North America and Canada appear to have a mixture of certified and non-certified dental assistants depending on the local requirements. Since mandatory registration in the UK in 2008, this is no longer permissible. When it comes to what is known in the UK as additional duties, and in Canada, for a level II dental nurse, primary qualifications are required and especially in Canada if intraoral work is to take place. This appears not to be the case in some states in North America. North America and Canada appear to have a much broader scope of practice, and both have a level of acceptance of unregulated dental assistants working within the field.

There remains some uncertainty for dental nurses in Canada and North America with regard to self-regulation and a lack of formal regulation. This has resulted in difficulty in fully establishing dental nursing as a profession. In addition, there is confusion as to what dental nurses can and cannot undertake across the states and provinces of these two countries.

An important variation that we see between the UK, North America and Canada is the matter of indemnity for dental nurses. In the latter two, the requirement for indemnity varies widely across the different states and provinces and is not always deemed necessary. This of course is not the case in the UK where all registered dental nurses must carry indemnity. It is a mandatory requirement for continued registration and must be declared in writing each year when registration is renewed. Working without indemnity would be likely to result in erasure from the register.

There is consensus for a number of skills and attributes of a dental nurse/assistant and they are noted as background knowledge; manual dexterity; co-ordination and proficiency in multiple significant skills aligned to delegable functions. Dental assistants/nurses are consistently recognised as 'critical' members of the dental team. After that, the commonalities become vaguer, as the procedures that dental nurses/assistants who are certified/regulated routinely perform when comparing North America, Canada and the UK are, in some cases, vastly different.

There is commonality in places of employment, although the UK has a very mixed workplace and has seen a shift from being predominantly NHS to having a stronger private market in primary care at least. In both North America and Canada, dental and oral care is predominantly provided through private plans. The common settings are:

- private practice with payment plans
- mixed practice
- NHS practice
- hospital setting
- community/salaried service
- public health
- secured settings
- corporate
- charitable provision
- educational facility – teaching
- educational facility – clinical assessment.

Republic of Ireland

Lynch et al. (2008) described the opinions and attitudes of dental nurses in Ireland to their roles and suitability of training, shortly after statutory registration had been introduced in the UK. They surveyed dental nurses via a postal questionnaire. The findings were that 'within the group of dental nurses surveyed, there was a lack of clarity surrounding their perception of their key duties. This could present challenges to the effective delivery of oral healthcare regimens within Ireland'.

In Ireland, the permitted duties of registered dental nurses include (Dental Council of Ireland 2001):

- providing assistance, short of the practice of dentistry, in the delivery of dental treatments
- preparation of surgeries for dental procedures;

- preparation and sterilisation of dental instruments and disinfection of equipment
- reception, patient welfare and health promotion.

Until the introduction of the Irish national training scheme, the primary dental nurse training programme in Ireland was the UK National Certificate Examination for Dental Nurses. The Irish national training scheme for dental nurses is a joint initiative between Dublin Dental University Hospital and Cork University Dental School and Hospital. Despite there being no requirement to have a dental qualification, high numbers of dental nurses take the qualification each year. Over recent years, two other providers have entered the dental nurse training landscape: Athlone Institute, which offers a BSc in Dental Practice Management with Oral Health Promotion, and Marion College, which offers the Level 6 Higher Certificate in Dental Nursing/Traineeship.

The Register of Dental Nurses in Ireland is a voluntary body. It is not mandatory to register as a dental nurse in order to practise in the Republic of Ireland. However, only registered dental nurses are permitted to take dental radiographs to the prescription of a dentist, having completed a Dental Council-approved course in dental radiography (Dental Council of Ireland 2021). The Dental Council of Ireland has produced a code of ethics and conduct for dental nurses.

Europe

Eaton et al. (2019) consider the variation in provision and cost of oral healthcare in 11 European countries. Included in their analysis is an interesting comment on provision of dental nursing. The paper reported that the role of dental nurses across these 11 countries varied widely.

In nine countries, if a dental nurse had additional training and there was a prescription from a dentist, they could take radiographs. In Germany it was reported that if the dental nurse had undertaken training in extended duties, they could perform supragingival scaling and polishing. In Denmark, after training, a dental nurse could place a filling under the supervision of a dentist and also perform supragingival scaling and polishing. In seven countries (Denmark, England, Germany, Ireland, Netherlands, Romania and Scotland), dental nurses were allowed to give oral hygiene instruction. In France, dental nurses are not allowed to perform any treatment within a treatment plan.

The paper considered where dental nurses assisted dentists and dental hygienists when they provided treatment. In nine countries (all except France, Poland and Romania), it was reported that the dentist would be assisted by a fully trained dental nurse. In France and Romania, dental nurses also acted as receptionists so may not be chairside all the time to assist. With the exception of Spain, dental hygienists either always or usually worked with a dental nurse to assist.

Finally, it was reported that the concept of team dentistry was not accepted in France and the authors posed the question of whether the lack of dental nurses influenced the quality of care in that country. As we can see, there is considerable variation in the roles and responsibilities for dental nurses across Europe.

Australia

Currently there are no qualification requirements for dental assistants in Australia and most are trained on the job. There are vocational qualifications that can be taken. The British Dental Journal Team (2021) interviewed dental nurses working in Australia and it was reported that there is no mandatory registration or continuing professional development requirement.

Worldwide

Roder (1978) reviewed the employment of dental nurses at that time and found that 29 countries employed dental nurses in a similar capacity to New Zealand school dental nurses: Australia, Brunei, Burma, Canada, Ceylon, Columbia, Costa Rica, Cuba, Ghana, Haiti, Hong Kong, Indonesia, Italy, Jamaica, Kenya, New Zealand, Nigeria, Papua New Guinea, Paraguay, Senegal, Sierre Leone, Sudan, Singapore, South Vietnam, Taiwan, Thailand, Uganda, United Kingdom and Zambia. In Pakistan an apprenticeship module training pathway is available and opportunities for promotion are reported to be good.

Whilst Roder (1978) writes about dental nurses undertaking a wide range of interventions, including restorations and extractions, it is likely that she is largely describing dental hygienists or dental therapists rather than dental nurses.

Roder discusses factors that favour the employment of dental nurses and one of the greatest factors is where there is a shortage of dentists. It seems at such times the utilisation of personnel who could be regarded as being quicker to train and cheaper to pay is a powerful incentive. Hobdell et al. (1975) stated that 'when there is a manpower shortage in a professional field, it is a well-established practice to assign simpler duties to auxiliaries, thereby reducing the burden on the fully trained'.

In South Africa, dental nurse training is full time in a university setting.

Nigeria introduced the first dental nursing examination in West Africa in 2021. Here dental nursing is a specialty division of nursing. The dental nurse is responsible for handling and managing oral healthcare. They work closely with dentists.

As we can see, there are many similarities in the evolution, roles and responsibilities of dental nursing across the world. However, there remain important differences in the actual work that can be undertaken, the training that is needed or available (initial and continuing) and whether individuals need to be registered or certified.

References

American Dental Assistants Association (ADAA) (2022). Available at: www.adaausa.org

BDJ Team (2021). Dental nurses around the world. *BDJ Team*, **8**, 32–33.

Canadian Dental Assistants Association (CDAA) (2022). Available at: www.cdaa.ca/da-promotion/?lang=en

Dental Council of Ireland (2001). Scheme for the establishment of a class of auxiliary dental worker to be known as Dental Nurse. Dental Council of Ireland, Dublin.

Dental Council of Ireland (2021). Use of ionising radiation for dental purposes. Available at: www.dentalcouncil.ie/g_ionisingradiation.php

Eaton, K.A., Ramsdale, M., Leggett, H., et al. (2019). Variations in the provision and cost of oral healthcare in 11 European countries: a case study. *International Dental Journal*, **69**, 130–140.

General Dental Council (2022). Registration reports. Available at: www.gdc-uk. org/about-us/what-we-do/the-registers/registration-reports

Hobdell, M.H., Burt, B.A., Longhurst, P. (1975). A method of planning a dental treatment program for an institutionalised population. *Community Dentistry and Oral Epidemiology*, 3(4), 166–173.

James, Y. (2016). *Building Capacity in Dental Assisting Research: The Self-Reported Impact of Occupational Health Stressors on the Work-Life of Canadian Dental Assistants*. Canadian Dental Assistants Association, Ottawa. Available at: www.cdaa.ca/cdaamedia/2016/05/BCDAR-Final-Report-2016.pdf

Lynch, C.D., O'Byrne, M.T., McConnell, R.J., Neville, P. (2008). Duties and training of dental nurses: how do Irish practices conform to European standards? *Community Dental Health*, 25, 98–102.

Moffat, S.M., Lyndie, A., Page, F., Thomson, W.M. (2017). New Zealand's school dental service over the decades; its response to social, political, and economic influences, and the effect on oral health inequalities. *Frontiers in Public Health*, 5, 1–18.

Oral Health Workforce Research Center (OHWRC) (2015). The Dental Assistant Workforce in the United States, 2015. Available at: https://oralhealthworkforce.org/wp-content/uploads/2015/11/Dental_Assistant_Workforce_2015.pdf

Reed, D. (2021). The history of dental nurses. *BDJ Team*, 8, 48–51.

Roder, D.M. (1978). The employment of dental nurses. *Journal of Public Health Dentistry*, 38, 159–171.

Thomson, T. (2015). *Shining a light on dental assistants*. MA thesis, McGill University. Available at: https://escholarship.mcgill.ca/concern/theses/fj236510g

Chapter 4 **Training and qualifications**

This chapter explores the range of clinical training and education available to dental nurses since the early days of the role in the UK. It will include formal and informal training providers. The impact of education for dental nurses will be linked to Chapters 5 and 7 and the role played in the emergence of dental nursing as a stand-alone profession within dentistry. The chapter will also review current qualifications that will appeal to dental nurses who wish to progress their career.

As has been established in earlier chapters, dental nursing, particularly in the UK, has seen a dramatic change in the last century. Other than the short period in which dental nurses were identified as dental dressers who carried out a range of dental activity under the supervision of a dentist (Gelbier 2006), the early dental nurses held the role of chaperone and administrator and were often a relative of the dentist. Any learning that transpired was on the job and in-house. By the 1940s, the formalisation of dental nurse training, known as dental assistants at the time, took its first landmark step in the UK, following the path of the North American states.

With the first examining board set up in 1943, dental nursing, as a recognised profession, began its journey. For many years, the first examination was an 'open access examination' (Sell 2005). In the earliest days the training was associated with the dental schools and later training was delivered at evening classes or in the practice, while some trainees were self-taught. It is worth noting that in 1964 the Voluntary National Register was established to encourage dental assistants to train and become qualified (BADN 2015). This of course was at a time when mandatory registration was not in place and when

How to Develop Your Career in Dental Nursing, First Edition. Edited by Janine Brooks and Fiona Ellwood.
© 2023 John Wiley & Sons Ltd. Published 2023 by John Wiley & Sons Ltd.

beyond the community and hospital settings, very little accountability was placed on the training provider. It is important to also acknowledge that dental nurse education and training were and continue to be delivered as part of the military. Whilst dental nurse students initially studied the military qualification, they now obtain the Diploma in dental nursing. Dental nursing in the military is explored further in Chapter 5. According to John et al. (2002), the dental nursing landscape was to be formally appraised as a result of the 1993 Nuffield Report.

In Oxford in 2002, a survey highlighted that of 254 responding dental nurses, only 101 had formal qualifications and 153 had no formal qualifications (John et al. 2002). A similar survey in Yorkshire in 2004 detailed 410 responding dental nurses, of which 246 held a dental nursing qualification and 164 had no formal dental nursing qualifications (Mercer et al. 2007). These findings echoed commentary by Lavery (cited in Sell 2005) making clear that the dental nursing awards and qualifications were optional and that there was much to do, heading into mandatory registration.

Professional registration and dental nurse qualifications

The introduction of mandatory General Dental Council (GDC) registration in 2008 changed the dental nursing landscape in the UK forever. Alongside mandatory registration (GDC 2008) came the requirement for awarding bodies of dental nursing qualifications to seek approval from the GDC. This had a ripple effect on the dental nurse training providers and in essence commanded measures of quality at every level and across every component of the provision. This raised the bar when it came to dental nurse training and also encapsulated the course content, formative assessment designs and endpoint assessment strategies. It was, of course, influenced by the GDC setting out the learning outcomes that needed to be met within the teaching and learning arena, and in the workplace (GDC 2015), as well as the requirement for specific areas of the curriculum to be assessed.

As part of these changes, the GDC developed an infrastructure that included an inspection framework, and which was aligned to the awarding body approval system. All approved courses were, and continue to be, inspected to ensure that quality provision of teaching, learning and assessment remains in place and the GDC requirements continue to be met. The intended outcome of these quality-driven measures was and is to ensure as far as reasonably possible that the dental nurse entering the GDC registration process meets the GDC requirement criteria of a 'safe beginner'.

Dental nursing qualifications

Putting the dental nursing qualifications into context with general education is not something that is generally considered, until a dental nurse decides to look beyond the role of dental nursing. Dental nursing is rarely a career that is alluded to in schools or colleges for those in full-time education or at education career events, unlike general nursing or dentistry. Educational qualifications are split into levels 1–8 in England, Wales and Northern Ireland and most qualifications have a 'difficulty' level. The higher the level, the more difficult the qualification is. A level 3 in England, Wales and Northern Ireland is equivalent to two A-levels, BTEC Nationals, International Baccalaureate and Advanced Apprenticeships. The level descriptors are not identical across the UK. England, Wales and Northern Ireland use the same level descriptors but Scotland uses a different system of levels, this is explored when discussing the Scottish Vocational Qualification later in this chapter.

It is important to recognise the historical perspective of dental nursing examinations in the UK as this helps to navigate what has become a busy landscape and fast-moving arena. The first National Certificate in the UK was developed by the National Examining Board for Dental Nurses and Assistants (NEBDNA). The early examination consisted of a written and oral examination, the first being held in 1943 and continued year on year, except in 1947–1948. As time moved on and roles expanded, the examination was adapted to include a practical section. For several years, the examination consisted of a choice of three out of four essay subjects, a viva and practical mixing test, as well as a spotter track of a hundred instruments. Alongside the numerous changes over time came name changes too and this has been discussed in Chapter 2. From here on, within this chapter, the examining board is referred to as the National Examining Board for Dental Nurses (NEBDN).

The day-to-day training for the NEBDN student requires hands-on vocational work in the dental workspace, supported by both informal and formal supervision and mentorship from those with dental expertise. The NEBDN gained approval from the GDC and has continued, since mandatory registration, to work in the dental nurse training space. The roles of the supervisor and mentor are now formalised within the NEBDN award and key to the NEBDN quality measures. The NEBDN approves and has oversight of all the NEBDN centres and has ultimate responsibility for their quality activity. It is worth noting that the NEBDN primary dental nursing award is the equivalent of a level 3 qualification.

In 2012 the NEBDN took the decision to update the National Certificate and the examination strategy; it also became known as the National Diploma in Dental Nursing. At the time of writing, the examination consists of a written and practical component, supported by on-the-job training and a record of experience log. The examination consists of two parts: 60 multiple-choice questions (MCQs), 40 extended matching questions (EMQs) and a range of objective structured clinical examination (OSCE) stations. Examinations are typically held three times a year and are divided into an OSCE examination and a written examination. The course is currently provided by a number of different types of providers, from dental school settings to private training providers, and can take between 12 and 24 months to complete. The bulk of the day-to-day learning continues to be work based. This also requires protected learning time in the workplace and a commitment from employers and other members of the team to contribute to the development and learning journey of the student dental nurse (GDC 2016).

The NEBDN was for many years the only National Certificate for dental nurses in the UK. In 2000, the awarding body City and Guilds introduced a National Vocational Qualification (NVQ) which was the first formal level 3 qualification for dental nurses in the UK. This was a huge turning point in dental nurse education, the qualification becoming assessment driven and with a central focus on work-based competence. What was being assessed was the ability to perform the practical skills and tasks required to undertake the job well. This qualification became known as the Level 3 Diploma in Dental Nursing.

The NVQ qualification required students to complete an extensive work-based portfolio and undertake a multiple-choice questions examination without a practical assessment. It placed greater demands on the workplace and existing team, relying more on professional judgements of skills routinely observed and collaborative working between the workplace and the training centre. This qualification has seen various adaptations and iterations over the years and has also adjusted to make effective and efficient use of modern technologies. In adopting this more formal approach to dental nurse education, it became plain that there was a need to train and employ a fit-for-purpose workforce to undertake the educational duties. In the case of the early NVQ, the educational workforce was made up of assessors, tutors, internal verifiers, external verifiers, examination invigilators and presiding examiners.

The current qualification awarded by City and Guilds is the level 3 Extended Diploma in Dental Nursing. The student must provide a portfolio of evidence which is judged as a pass/fail, produce at least five observations of practice and two of those must be witnessed by an assessor. A further observation is undertaken by an independent assessor as part of the end-point assessment and the student must successfully complete an online multiple-choice examination consisting of 45 questions over 90 minutes, with a common completion time for the whole course of 14–18 months.

The introduction of the NVQ appeared to open the door for further dental nursing qualifications to come to fruition; qualifications from level 3 up to degree level have centre stage in dental nursing training, all with differing entry requirements, and some provide a wider opportunity to progress within both dentistry and allied professions. The nation-specific qualifications for Wales and Scotland have been welcomed within the nations and they appeal specifically because they lend themselves to the variations of guidance set out by local government decisions and drivers, and the Welsh qualifications are available in the Welsh language.

The Council for Awards in Care, Health and Education (CACHE) was approved in 2015 to provide a level 3 Diploma in Principles and Practice of Dental Nursing (QCF). This qualification has evolved to follow the apprenticeship framework. The teaching, learning and outcomes are again set and guided by the GDC approval system, seeking the safe beginner in successful dental nurses. The qualification is not dissimilar to the other dental nursing qualifications. It uses a range of assessment methods and includes direct observation by an assessor from the training centre, professional discussions and reflective accounts in a reflective log, questions and the completion of a task assessment for knowledge learning outcomes. This course gives 49 credits at level 3 with a usual duration of 12–18 months for completion.

Scotland and Wales have both developed qualifications based upon the apprenticeship framework, with the content and assessment methods mapped to the Scottish Credit and Qualifications Framework (SCQF) and Qualifications Wales (QW) respectively. Minor adjustments have been made in the content that are specific to the nation requirements, and both are funded by their local governments. Both nations have level 3 qualifications; Wales also has a level 4 qualification at the time of writing, and both are available in the Welsh language. The level 4 qualification has a more in-depth approach and is intended to be part of an escalation pathway to other dental qualifications if the student wishes to progress.

The Scotland system is different, as previously noted. The SVQ level 3 is recognised as a SCQF level 7 qualification. Scotland also has the Higher National Certificate (HNC) in dental nursing awarded at SCQF level 7 and the Higher National Diploma (HND) (level 8) which builds on the primary qualification. They also have a Bachelor of Science degree (BSc) level 9 programme for dental nurses which is their penultimate qualification for dental nurses. This requires individuals to already hold the primary qualification and is awarded by the West of Scotland University, delivered through New College Lanarkshire.

The University of Northampton was the first to be approved by the GDC to award a foundation degree. The programme is a two-year full-time level 5 course and the modules reflect 20 credits each, with one module in each semester affording 60 credits. This course has a strong focus on linking theory to practice and is delivered to level 4 at stage 1 and level 5 at stage 2; at stage 2 there is a strong focus on research and advanced work-based learning. As a higher-level qualification, inevitably there is an entry requirement, currently of DD at A-level or a level 3 NVQ. The assessment methods include an examination, viva voce, clinical simulation tests, presentations, assignments and the completion of a clinical portfolio. Despite being a higher-level qualification, the course follows the same learning outcomes set by the GDC for all dental nursing qualifications but requires a deeper level of educational skills from the student. The increased level of the course is still confined to the same scope of practice for all dental nurses but brings a different suite of transferable skills to the fore.

The Universities of Portsmouth and Teesside both offer Certificates in Higher Education (level 4) in dental nursing. Both are one-year courses leading to registration. These qualifications appear to make the transition to dental hygiene and/or dental therapy more accessible. The Certificate in Higher Education in dental nursing is entered through the Universities and Colleges Admissions Service (UCAS) tariff point system, although mature students are considered with equivalent qualifications. The successful students are awarded a total of 120 credits. The University of Portsmouth offers this course on a full-time or part-time basis and suggests that earning capacity and opportunities are greater on successful completion of the Higher Education Certificate. Students are assessed through reflection logs, practical skills, oral and practical examinations and written assignments.

The University of Portsmouth also offers a BSc (Hons) in Advanced Dental Nursing. This is an undergraduate qualification, taking three years to complete; at the end of year 1, successful students can apply to become GDC registrants. Students completing the BSc qualification have gone on to take up research, teaching and Masters programmes.

The new T-level qualifications were launched in September 2020. T-levels are two-year courses which are taken after GCSEs and are broadly equivalent to three A-Levels. The courses have been developed in collaboration with employers and education providers. The content is designed to meet the needs of industry and prepares students for entry into skilled employment, an apprenticeship or related technical study through further or higher education. Not dissimilar to the widening participation agenda, but with the emphasis being on core content, to include sciences and reflect the needs of the health and science sector. Notably, these qualifications are England centric and aimed at 16–18 year olds. They are an alternative to A-levels. The qualifications are being gradually rolled out, with the first three T-levels available in September 2020, a further seven in September

2021, six in September 2022 and the remaining seven in September 2023. The Education and Skills Funding Agency provides guidance specific to dental nursing and T-level delivery (E&SFA 2022).

T-levels are a new way of learning and gaining a dental nursing qualification, and have been heralded as a landmark 'revolution in technical education' (NCFE 2020). Some are considering this as a escalator route through dental nursing and on into dental hygiene and therapy. From 2022, the Northern Council for Further Education (NCFE) plans to offer the first T-level occupational specialism in dental nursing.

In October 2022, a small number of senior dental nurses were accepted onto the level 6 programme at Keele University, to undertake the Advanced Clinical Practitioner Apprenticeship qualification. This is a new pathway and not one that has been open to dental nurses before. It is, however, being readily embraced by members of the wider health sector. Given the nature of the course, it is likely to attract huge demand, but only a few will be able to apply for the course currently, simply because of the level of autonomy required. This course is shouting out to those dental nurses in secondary and community care settings and especially those managing teams and clinics. This must be recognised as a huge step forward in many ways.

Additional duties

It was noted in Chapter 2 that postcertification awards were prominent in 1989 and provided predominantly by the NEBDN. The early postcertificate awards were Oral Health Education, Dental Sedation Nursing, Special Care Dental Nursing and Orthodontic Dental Nursing, followed by Dental Radiography, and all have been deemed to be the equivalent of a level 4 qualification. Since mandatory registration, further postcertification awards have been adopted by the NEBDN: Dental Implant Nursing and Fluoride Varnish Application. In addition to this, other training providers now deliver postcertificate awards; for example, the British Dental Association awards the Oral Health Certificate and Dental Radiography, as do a number of dental schools.

Mandatory registration brought with it a wider range of allowable skill sets seen through the lens of additional duties and an explosion

Table 4.1 Additional duties, adapted from GDC Scope of Practice document.

Intra- and extraoral photography	Placing rubber dam	Repairing the acrylic component of removable appliances
Pouring, casting and trimming models	Measuring and recording plaque indices	Applying topical anaesthetic to the prescription of a dentist
Shade taking	Removing sutures after the wound has been checked by a dentist	Constructing mouthguards and bleaching trays to the prescription of a dentist
Tracing cephalographs	Constructing occlusal registration rims and special trays	Constructing vacuum-formed retainers to the prescription of a dentist
Taking impressions to the prescription of a dentist or clinical dental technician (where appropriate)	Applying fluoride varnish either on prescription from a dentist or direct as part of a structured dental health programme	

of newly designed courses (Table 4.1). These skills are carried out on prescription from, or under the direction of, another registrant (GDC 2013).

Impact of registration and education

Reflecting upon the earlier works of John et al. (2002) and Ross and Ibbetson (2006) prior to implementation of mandatory registration and educational qualifications, the envisaged impacts suggested that forging professional registration on the back of educational attainment could add to existing recruitment problems, place greater demands on training providers and require a broader provision of training centres. Once qualified and registered, the requirements of continuing professional development and lifelong learning would bring a different set of challenges, despite being seen as raising the profile and status of the dental nurse. Ross (cited in Sell 2005 p.18) had previously suggested that UK dental nurses upon registration would '. . . move along the medical model . . . alluding to nurse practitioners, nurse consultants and nurse specialists'.

The complexity of the transition period was not to be underestimated. For those already employed as a dental nurse, navigating the options appeared far from straightforward. For those holding the National Certificate upon successfully registering with the GDC, former titles were superseded, and they became known as dental nurses as part of the two-year introductory window (also known as mediated entry). It goes without saying that this community of dental nurses faced the most change and showed excitement, hesitation and resilience towards mandatory registration and everything that would accompany it.

Dental nurse students post-2008, taking up the baton of becoming the first generation working to statutory requirements from the onset, started in a very different place and with the expectations of having to train, demonstrate competence and, on successful completion of an approved course, applying to join the GDC professional register. They did this knowing that being a registered dental nurse would include the undertaking of continuing professional development (CPD) and life-long learning. This could be identified as the beginning of the modernisation of the world of dental nursing, as well as the heightening of the awareness and profile of the dental nurse as a professional.

After implementation of mandatory registration and qualifications but prior to the new ECPD scheme of 2017, Turner et al. (2012) established through research that some dental nurses had reported a greater sense of professionalism and respect, and with this had come greater responsibility. Conversely, others reported financial challenges aligned to qualifications and CPD, as well as the annual retention fee and increased pressures on personal time to undertake CPD as negative elements of being a registrant. Also, many dental nurses reported that further education through the medium of CPD did not help them do their job better or gain the support of their employers. Sadly, it appears that the negative responses collated by Turner et al. (2012) have now become the instruments behind the exodus of dental nurses from the profession over more recent years, not helped by the impact of the COVID-19 pandemic. This brings into focus the strong question of career motivation, which will be considered in Chapter 5.

The research undertaken by Turner et al. (2012) indicates that dental nurses were, in general, keen to progress and undertake additional courses and duties and this of course goes hand in hand with CPD requirements and a need to ensure that educational providers are aligned to the GDC provider guidelines (GDC 2018a). This relies on the registrant to make wise decisions before engaging in learning. The only exception is the flexibility to make effective use of the GDC mapping document (GDC 2018b) if, for instance, a university certificate does not meet the requirements of the GDC certificate, yet a registrant believes the learning is worthy of CPD recognition.

Given the enormous breadth of qualification, knowledge, skills and behaviours, it is perhaps pertinent to take a moment here to consider the transferable skills of the dental nurse, especially given the recent climate of the pandemic. Sadly, dental nurses were not granted a list of transferable competencies in England as can be seen within the Standard Operating Procedures version 2 (20 April 2020). The picture did differ across the nations and seemed to cause a barrier to the masses who desperately wanted to lean in and do more. The transferable competencies in England were outlined as follows.

- Identify, assess and manage medical emergencies.
- Implement, perform and manage effective decontamination and infection control according to current guidelines.
- Recognise the signs of abuse or neglect in vulnerable groups and local procedures that should be followed when reporting such circumstances.

Those within the secondary care and community settings worked to the requirements and demands of their workplace and in some cases were redeployed, although the sensitive topic of delivering vaccines remained. Dental nurses in the secondary care and community settings have a different set of skills and were able to do more with ease. Perhaps the time has now come for those who can, to take this long-standing battle on and carve out a pathway. A pathway that is an enabler for secondary care dental nursing members, whilst looking closely at the gaps between primary and secondary care with an intention of creating an educational bridge. It is time for the so-called 'can do' approach.

Continuing professional development (CPD)

It is important that the introduction of CPD is now addressed. CPD has been perceived as a mechanism for maintaining high standards of care and current ethical professional practice through education and learning. It is against this backdrop that the GDC incorporated the requirement to undertake CPD on an annual basis and across a five-year cycle. This was a requirement of remaining on the regulatory professional register and very much a component of the journey to registration for dental nurses. The initial CPD framework (Table 4.2) was updated in 2017 and introduced in 2018, as shown in Table 4.3.

The initial CPD requirement took a global view of dental care professionals and followed the design for dental practitioners, although the hours were different and the CPD cycle dates differed. Despite the number of hours being identified as the minimum number of hours, it became apparent that this was perceived by many registrants as the actual number of hours.

Table 4.2 Initial CPD requirements adapted from GDC (2008).

Professional group (2008)	Number of hours	Verifiable	Non-verifiable	CPD year date
Dentists	250	75	175	1 January–31 December
All dental care professionals	150	50	100	1 August–31 July

Table 4.3 Current CPD requirements adapted from GDC (2017).

Professional group (2017)	Number of verifiable hours	CPD year date
Dentists	Minimum 100	1 January–31 December
Dentists (temporary registrants)	Minimum 20	1 January–31 December
Dental therapist, dental hygienist, orthodontic therapists, clinical dental technician	Minimum 75	1 August–31 July
Dental nurses and dental technicians	Minimum 50	1 August–31 July

As is reflected in Table 4.2, the initial GDC CPD scheme (2008) required all dental care professionals to undertake both verifiable and non-verifiable CPD. Each registrant was required to make an annual declaration of their CPD undertakings, their indemnity provision and eventually their commitment to equality, diversity and inclusion. The hours were identified as minimum hours to be accrued over a five-year cycle. The initial scheme identified core CPD topics of:

- medical emergencies 10 hours
- disinfection and decontamination five hours
- radiography and radiation safety five hours.

Recommendations were also for the registrant to remain up to date on the following subjects.

- Legal issues and ethics.
- Complaints handling.
- Oral cancer.
- Safeguarding of children/young people and vulnerable adults.

The updated CPD scheme refers to the same topics and number of hours but there is a slight change of the language whereby all the topics are now seen as recommended and dental professionals must undertake CPD topics that firstly align to their day-to-day activity and to any future fields of activity as well as fields of interest. In effect, if a dental nurse has a number of roles, perhaps mixing clinical with non-clinical, then they need to maintain and update each of those areas within each cycle.

Figure 4.1 reflects the updated ECPD scheme (2018a) which outlines the required CPD hours for all registrants and a further separation of the registrant groups, meaning dental nurses and dental technicians are required to complete a minimum of 50 hours of CPD whilst the other non-dentist groups are required to undertake a minimum of 75 hours. There is no longer a requirement to declare non-verifiable CPD. There is, however, a greater emphasis on reflective practice, designing CPD activity related to the individual's day-to-day activity and a requirement to undertake a minimum of 10 hours of CPD every two years. In addition to this, the GDC has made clear that a practitioner can decide to not undertake CPD in any given year, but this must be recorded as 0 hours in the annual declaration (GDC 2018a).

All learning and CPD must also be mapped to at least one of the GDC development outcomes which are classified as shown in Table 4.4.

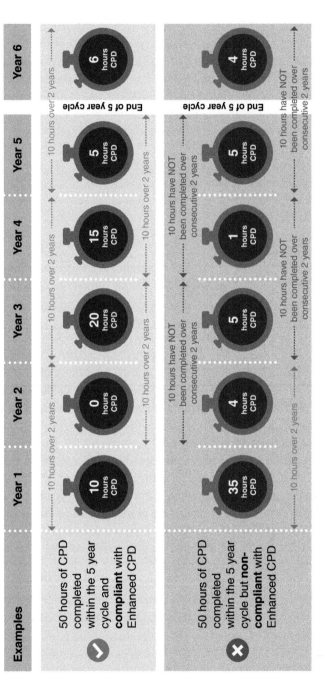

Figure 4.1 Updated ECPD scheme. Source: General Dental Council 2018a/General Dental Council.

Table 4.4 GDC development outcomes.

A	Effective communication with patients, the dental team and others across dentistry, including when obtaining consent, dealing with complaints, and raising concerns when patients are at risk
B	Effective management of self and effective management of others or effective work with others in the dental team, in the interests of patients; providing constructive leadership where appropriate
C	Maintenance and development of knowledge and skill within your field of practice
D	Maintenance of skills, behaviours and attitudes which maintain patient confidence in you and the dental profession and put patients' interests first

Source: General Dental Council 2018a/General Dental Council.

Education providers are required to ensure their training meets the requirements of the GDC and certificates produced for registrants must include aims, objectives, learning outcomes and which of the development outcomes the training covers.

Reflective practitioner

This sea change in personal development has, however, seen the emergence of the reflective practitioner. According to Johns (2022, p.1), reflection is a skill, an art and a craft if it is undertaken well. Johns refers to it as 'professional artistry'. All GDC registrants, inclusive of dental nurses, are expected to reflect periodically on their ECPD activity, not only showing learning but how the learning can inform their practice and in particular benefit patients. The reflective activity is also identified as a means of informing future learning and training needs and contributing to the concept of life-long learning and the development of personal development plans. Johns (2022, p.3) asserts that 'reflection is a process of self-inquiry towards self-realisation'. It is clear that reflection and reflective practice take on many guises, but how and when such skills are introduced to dental nurses is far from clear.

Despite this, the GDC asserts that becoming a reflective practitioner is both important and beneficial and as a result, has outlined its views and requirements for reflection (GDC 2019). It suggests that 'reflection foster[s] improvements in practice and services', and that reflection 'provides a basis by which resilience can be acquired, wellbeing improved, and professional commitment deepened' (GDC 2019). Against this premise, reflective practice perhaps should be an essential skill that is both taught and acquired throughout primary dental nursing qualifications and continually revisited and facilitated as an ongoing GDC registrant.

At one level it is possible to see the context in which the registrant as a reflective practitioner has come to fruition, but becoming a reflective practitioner is a skill that goes beyond the application of any model and habitual practice. Becoming a reflective practitioner brings insight and clarity, it goes beyond description to inquiry of self and celebrates being curious. Loori (2005) frames curiosity as a way of opening up possibilities and paying attention to what we truly see, as only then can we begin to reflect. None of this is to deny that reflection has a place in learning and informing change, but it is clear that reflection and reflective practice are far from straightforward. They can be subjective and despite being individual, it often takes collective actions to have insight and for change to occur. For those who feel uncertain about reflection and reflective writing, it can be helpful at the beginning to work with a mentor who can guide and support the process until you feel confident to 'go it alone'.

The notion of being individual adds to the growing identity of self as a dental nurse and the concepts of professionality and professional identity. According to Evans (2008, p.25), professionality is 'the singular unit of professionalism', whereas professional identity is identified as a set of attributes that characterise specific groups of people. In searching for a new identity as part of the rapidly evolving dental nursing landscape, it cannot be assumed that there is one and perhaps in this time of change and opportunity the dental nursing profession can write its own professional narrative. This will be addressed within Chapter 5 as we focus on twenty-first century skills and the future of dentistry.

References

British Association of Dental Nurses (BADN) (2015). The Founding of BADN. Available at: www.nature.com/articles/bdjteam201588
Education and Skills Funding Agency (E&SFA) (2002). Annex J. T Level Technical Qualification in Health – guidance specific to dental nursing.

Available at: https://assets.publishing.service.gov.uk/government/uploads/ system/uploads/attachment_data/file/1064102/Annex_J_Dental_ Nursing_Industry_Placement_Guidance.pdf

Evans, L. (2008). Professionalism, professionality and the development of education professionals. *British Journal of Educational Studies*, **56**(1). 20–38.

Gelbier, S. (2006). Dental dressers: 1920–1942. *Dental Historian*, **46**, 27–46.

General Dental Council (GDC) (2008). Previous CPD Scheme. Available at: www.gdc-uk.org/education-cpd/cpd/cpd-scheme-2008-2017

General Dental Council (GDC) (2015). Preparing for Practice, revised edition. Available at: www.gdc-uk.org/docs/default-source/quality-assurance/ preparing-for-practice-(revised-2015).pdf

General Dental Council (GDC) (2016.) Student Professionalism and fitness to practise – what do you need to know? Available at : www.gdc-uk.org/ docs/default-source/guidance-for-students/student-professionalism-and- fitness-to-practise-an-introduction-for-students.pdf?sfvrsn=d34ea419_2

General Dental Council (GDC) (2017). Enhanced CPD guidance for professionals. Available at: www.gdc-uk.org/education-cpd/cpd/enhanced-cpd- scheme-2018

General Dental Council (GDC) (2018a). Enhanced CPD Scheme requirements. Available at: www.gdc-uk.org/education-cpd/cpd/enhanced-cpd- scheme-2018

General Dental Council (GDC) (2018b). Mapping document for verifiable CPD. Available at : https://view.officeapps.live.com/op/view.aspx?src= https%3A%2F%2Fwww.gdc-uk.org%2Fdocs%2Fdefault-source %2Fenhanced-cpd-scheme-2018%2Fmapping-document-for-verifiable- cpd.docx%3Fsfvrsn%3D7dde5584_2&wdOrigin=BROWSELINK

General Dental Council (GDC) (2019). Benefits of becoming a reflective practitioner – joint statement. Available at: www.nebdn.org/gdc-release- joint-statement-on-benefits-of-being-a-reflective-practitioner/

John, J.H., Thomas D., Richards, D., Evans, C. (2002). Regulating dental nurses in the UK. *British Dental Journal*, **193**, 207–209.

Johns, C. (2022). *Becoming a Reflective Practitioner*, 6th edn. John Wiley & Sons, Oxford.

Loori, J. (2005). *The Zen of Creativity: Cultivating Your Artistic Life*. Ballentine Books, New York.

Mercer, P., Bailey, H., Cook, P. (2007). Perceptions, attitudes and opinions of general dental practitioners and dental nurses to the provision of lifelong learning for the dental team. *British Dental Journal*, **202**, 747–753.

Northern Council for Further Education (NCFE) (2020.) T-levels. Available at: www.ncfe.org.uk/technical-education/t-levels/

Ross, M.K., Ibbetson, R.J. (2006). Educational needs and employment status of Scottish dental nurses. *British Dental Journal*, **201**, 661–666.

Sell C. (2005). History of PCDs: The rise and rise of PCDs. Available at: www.nature.com/articles/vital310.pdf

Turner, S., Ross, M.K., Ibbetson, R. (2012). The impact of registration and CPD on dental nurses. *Vital*, **9**(4), 24–31.

Chapter 5 **Career development**

This chapter will consider career development and opportunities for dental nurses at the time of writing. It will pick up the postregistration work, previously noted in Chapter 4, as postcertification work and examine the opportunities on the back of achieving those awards and qualifications, and look at career planning and portfolio building.

Career choices and developments are not new to dentistry but are often seen to be new to the field of dental nursing. There has certainly been a shift of minds since mandatory registration was introduced. This is not to ignore those who prior to this period made career choices and successfully achieved personal goals.

Historical perspectives of career development are associated with a need to classify people and place them into occupations. According to Brown and Brooks (2002), this was then linked to a person's status, earnings, wealth and lifestyle. Nevertheless, dental nurses have to date not always considered career development and choices. According to a survey conducted by the Society of British Dental Nurses in 2019, many dental nurses reported that there was no clear career pathway and little support for those who wished to progress, despite having taken additional awards. This has also been reflected in earlier works by Ross and Ibbetson (2006) and Mercer et al. (2007).

This does raise an interesting question as to how to define career progression. Is it an increase in responsibility, an increase in financial return or a more senior title? Is career progression about the job or about the person? Perhaps the easiest answer is that it is about both. Here are a few examples of activities that could be deemed as career progression.

How to Develop Your Career in Dental Nursing, First Edition. Edited by Janine Brooks and Fiona Ellwood.
© 2023 John Wiley & Sons Ltd. Published 2023 by John Wiley & Sons Ltd.

- Continuing professional education – gaining more qualifications and training.
- Joining a professional organisation – this can bring important networking opportunities, and exposure to strategic and political activities.
- Research – this could start small by undertaking audits in the practice or developing a patient engagement survey.
- Increased duties and responsibilities – perhaps taking on a lead role in the practice.
- Job assignments – introducing a new system into the practice.
- Supervising and supporting new members of staff.

These are all examples of developing yourself, developing your career. You don't have to take a qualification and examinations to be on a career pathway. Some of the above may attract increased financial remuneration, but all will add to your feelings of achievement and self-worth. The direction your career takes is personal to you and in most cases needs to be planned by yourself. Working with a mentor or a coach can help you to think more clearly what you would like to do. It's worth remembering that a career does not have to be a straight pathway from A to B. Of course, it also depends on what you define as B – what is the end goal? Many careers tack around, sometimes taking diversions, sometimes looping. Is your career all about the destination or is it more about the journey? Maybe lack of a career pathway is more about lack of career development.

Perkins (2019) describes how to develop a simple three-part script which describes your professional past, present and future self. Here is an example.

1. **Where have you been?** After completing my qualification, I started work at Park Lane dental practice. One highlight was introducing a new patient information brochure.
2. **Where are you now?** Since moving to Deanside Corporate, I've held the position of treatment co-ordinator and also taken the lead in induction and training for new dental nurses. I'm inspired to think about taking a further qualification as I really enjoy the engagement with patients and the educational side of dental nursing.
3. **Where are you (ideally) going?** I want to build on my skills. I'm really interested in expanding my role and I'm very motivated to . . .

This script is a helpful way to consolidate what you have and where you have skills. It will help you to think about the future, the next few years and what you would like to do. It is similar to a personal development plan (PDP), except it probably has a further vision than one year. Your PDP would complement the script, particularly if your future plans will take a little time to achieve.

Many dental nurses join the profession directly from full-time education and have given little thought to career progression. Whilst self-interest appears to be a factor in any notable progression, there appears to be little protected or supported time to develop such interests, open dialogue or feedback from peers or mentors that could help inform career choices. Progression of course means different things to different people, as does the context in which progression is both discussed and identified. Often the needs and demands of the population or workplace setting become drivers for dental employers to encourage specific career decisions for dental nurses rather than dental nurses taking control of their own career plans.

External drivers such as dental and oral disease patterns and trends, research advancement and advancement in technologies, techniques and materials are also influencers from the perspective of both the employer and the dental nurse. Here the dental nurse can begin to construct and shape their development, but not without constraints and limitations. Dental nurses need to become active agents in their career choices and decision making, but with this must come a desire to work differently and with buy-in from the whole profession. This means being future focused, understanding the philosophy of a career and how to design a career framework, so that talents can be nurtured and strengthened, and opportunity created.

This requires a great deal of thought, discussion and planning as dental nurses are often hampered by lack of autonomy in the workplace and the limitations placed upon them by the regulators, which links back to the Dentists' Act 1984. What is possible is to look at existing models of working and then move to models of working differently. One certainty is that both lifelong learning and thinking outside the box need to feature. Career management is perhaps new to many but is key to taking control and setting goals. Three broad factors are important on this journey.

1. To have a clear understanding of self.
2. To understand the dental landscape and opportunities.
3. To understand the conditions of success.

Clear understanding of self

Having a clear understanding of self helps to formulate focal points from which the locus of control can be taken, and career management can begin. Recognising one's aptitudes, abilities, interests, ambitions and limitations is a good starting point. Using a personality test may also prove to be effective on this journey of understanding self, for example the Myers–Briggs Type Indicator (www.myersbriggs.org/my-mbti-personality-type/mbti-basics/) or the DISC personal assessment tool (www.discprofile.com). Another effective tool which could support dental nurses is the SWOT analysis which looks beyond an individual's strengths and weaknesses and considers both opportunities and potential threats. Discovering who you really are, what your talents are and where your passion and enthusiasm lies can contribute to achieving professional satisfaction.

Knowledge of the dental landscape

Having a clear understanding of the dental landscape and allied fields helps dental nurses explore much broader options. Connecting with professional colleagues with an enquiring and creative mind will help to formulate interests and possibilities. A suggested tool here is the Thought Shower, a group problem-solving technique. The term was created by Henry McDonald in 2005 when he was Ireland editor of The Observer, to replace 'brain storming' (Osborn 1953). Having looked inwards and discovered more about 'self', this exercise is likely to be beneficial in exploring the dental arena and where dental nurses can best fit. It may be that something as simple as reshaping your existing role could set you off on a different trajectory, looking for training opportunities in specific fields and with different or better career outcomes and a greater sense of accomplishment.

Conditions of success

Arthur et al. (2005) defined career success 'as the accomplishment of desirable work-related outcomes at any point in a person's work experience over time' (p.179). Traditionally, the measures of success have been employment stability and salary but according to Shockley et al. (2016), these are not the only considerations for the modern employee. This appears to be echoed in the world of dental nursing whereby recognition, reward, opportunity and being valued contribute towards the notion of successful careers and career satisfaction of the modern-day dental nurse.

In previous chapters a range of primary qualifications for dental nurses have been identified, as well as the additional duties, awards and qualifications available once a dental nurse has become a GDC registrant. There are also a number of non-clinical awards and qualifications that are open to dental nurses which should be considered if there is to be a full and comprehensive view of the dental nursing landscape. What must also be included is the context and setting in which dental nurses are employed. One of the greatest challenges often presented is the mismatch between service need and the dental nurse's career ambition. Roles within the hospital and military setting are looked at separately.

Figure 5.1 presents a current but more traditional set of career opportunities, through additional qualifications, further training and successful application to the GDC registration process for a dental nurse. It demonstrates a mix of skill growth within the profession of

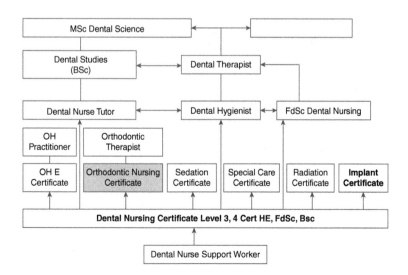

Figure 5.1 Dental nurse clinical opportunities.

dental nursing in addition to an escalator to other professional groups within the family of dentistry. This is not meant to be a complete picture but an indication of opportunities.

Lead roles

Figure 5.2 presents an overview of the lead clinical roles which have evolved in many primary care, community and corporate settings. Previously, most of these were core foundations of practice in the secondary care setting. Taking a lead role means working with stakeholders, creating policy, designing of workloads and ensuring high quality and standards are adhered to, as well as managing difficulties, risks and errors in a coherent and transparent manner. These roles require skills of leadership and management in addition to the substance of the lead role, for example, senior knowledge of implants, infection prevention, etc. twinned with acquired knowledge of how to lead and manage that particular specialist area.

Lead roles are also identified as 'champion' roles.

- *Oral health lead* – this role includes setting, planning and negotiating oral health strategies and their application through oral health team members. The key directive comes from the Delivering Better Oral Health toolkit (Office for Health Improvement and

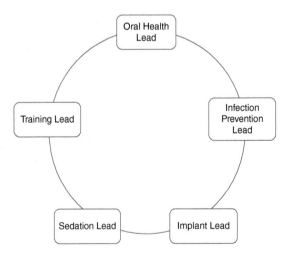

Figure 5.2 Lead clinical roles in primary care.

Disparities 2021) and NICE guidelines (2015). The general focus looks at population-level delivery rather than one-to-one delivery for better patient outcomes. In the dental setting the one-to-one approach is prominent but being part of oral health and public health teams appeals to many dental nurses. Much of this work currently sits within the community setting or within the local authority. This work also gives rise to working privately but with support and guidance, this can take you into care homes, allied healthcare training, schools and mother and toddler groups, to name but a few. There are a range of courses and public health courses that are relevant to this field.

- *Infection prevention and control (IPC) lead* – commonly takes control of all IPC matters and ensures all settings and individuals are aware of the most recent guidance and are applying it safely in the dental workplace. Individuals are responsible for the dissemination of up-to-date guidance and any changes and are likely to be involved in the auditing and reporting processes. They must keep up to date and maintain their CPD in line with the GDC guidelines. There are a range of courses aimed at IPC leads and leadership and IPC.

- *Implant lead nurses* – direct and guide the implant team and ensure all procedures run smoothly; they ensure learning is clearly distributed and that patients are kept well informed. Implant leads often work with the team co-ordinator and manage patients collectively. All implant leads must be current and up to date in dental procedures and maintain their skills in line with the GDC CPD guidelines. There are recognised training courses for implant leads.

- *Sedation lead* – the sedation lead has a shared responsibility to ensure that the team are trained and skilled and that all equipment is working and fit for purpose. They ensure that all required and necessary drugs are available and relevant stocks are in place. They ensure the patient is well informed, has followed all the guidance given and has consented to the treatment and procedure and reconfirms this. They also ensure everything is in place for patient recovery and are flexible to manage any changes of plan or emergency. Risk assessment is a key feature of this role. Formal training is available for dental nurses. Whilst this work is carried out in general practice, it is also carried out in the secondary care setting. General anaesthesia is a hospital provision (secondary care) and so dental nurses would be looking to move to that setting if this was a career choice.

- *Training lead* – the training lead co-ordinates all learning needs and provision in the dental setting and is often responsible for writing business cases. Other components of this role focus around providing training and keeping all team members up to date. The lead works with external providers and arranges training sessions and co-ordinates diaries. In some instances, the training lead collates and monitors the team's annual CPD and flags shortfalls. Depending on the size of the business, the training lead may be responsible for visiting numerous sites to deliver training and develop appropriate resources. This is a role that requires experience of training and education, being able to engage with mixed audiences and having an understanding of modern technologies.

Figure 5.3 gives a global view of some of the many non-clinical roles. Many of these roles form part of the more modern world of dental nursing and the dentistry arena today.

Treatment co-ordination is a thriving role born out of one-to-one consultations with patients. The treatment co-ordinator is often a dental nurse who has an exceptional knowledge base of any potential

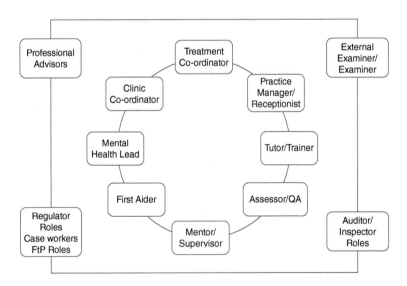

Figure 5.3 Non-clinical and academic roles.

treatments and can showcase and elevate casework and engage with clients. The treatment co-ordinator works closely with the dental surgeon to explain and inform patients about the options that are on offer for the treatment they require. According to Horton (2010), the treatment co-ordinator manages the treatment journey and choices of the client from start to finish and is often the first point of contact. They have time to listen to concerns, answer any questions and enhance the whole treatment and care experience. These roles are currently more prominent in private dental settings but are becoming more popular in mixed practice settings too and are certainly leading the way when it comes to new methods of working in modern-day dentistry.

The treatment co-ordinator role is designed to remove as much of the non-clinical work from the dentist as possible; a key intention is to change perceptions about dentistry and increase the uptake of treatments. Once clients have decided to go ahead with treatments and their experience is a positive one, they are more likely to stay with the practice. The treatment co-ordinator is responsible for new business and new clients bring new business. According to Horton (2010), the follow-through and uptake of treatments needs to be a key performance indicator, and this is why new client inquiries should be directed to the treatment co-ordinator.

The role is not about 'selling' dentistry – dentistry is a profession, not a 'shop'. It is about giving patients all the information they need to make treatment decisions and decide what is best for them in a more relaxed environment than the dental surgery. Dental nurses clearly have the advantage over a co-ordinator who does not have a clinical background.

Treatment co-ordinators need to be team players but must also work well on their own and be efficient. The ability to build a good rapport is essential given that all the preliminary work is undertaken by the treatment co-ordinator. Only when the patient wishes to know their suitability for treatments do they see the dentist. The treatment co-ordinator, if qualified and trained in specific procedures, can prepare all the clinical photographs and prescribed radiographs and upload everything ahead of the client visit. They also take on appointment scheduling and financial arrangements. Interestingly but perhaps not unexpectedly, treatment co-ordinators suggest that they are on performance-related pay. We could ponder how that might sit comfortably with putting patients' interests first. There are a number of providers offering treatment co-ordinator courses, and some use the term 'care co-ordinator'. At the time of writing the courses appear to be the equivalent of a level 3.

Administrative roles such as practice management and receptionist duties vary. Many dental nurses have dual roles, which include dental nursing and practice management. Whilst no formal register is held for practice managers or receptionists, training for the roles is essential. The duties can vary from setting to setting and are often dependent on the size of the business and patient groups. There are formal practice management qualifications ranging from level 4 up to degree level and some dental settings support dental nurses to undertake these. Practice management roles benefit from having attributes and skills such as being able to think and act strategically, being able to make informed, evidence-based decisions, being able to motivate team members, creating and maintaining an open and transparent culture, understanding organisational strategic direction and planning. Beyond this, effective interpersonal skills, communication and listening skills make the difference between a good practice manager/receptionist and a great one. Not all managers are given budgetary controls but having financial management skills is advantageous and leadership skills too. Leadership in itself is quite a complex field, but well worth exploring, if only to add further tools to your own profile.

Educational roles generate much interest but often receive the least amount of support and recognition. However, roles within some of the educational settings associated with the quality parameters are clearly defined and are set against educational foundations and structures. For those considering teaching, it is recommended that a minimum of a postgraduate certificate in education is achieved to create the maximum opportunities as a tutor/lecturer. Qualifications are available at a lower level, but they will limit teaching roles to further education and private education settings or their equivalent. These skills must also be part of any annual CPD planning if they make up a dental nurse's regular work activity. Teaching and assessing courses are very accessible and available online and span across a range of academic levels.

Teaching roles can be full time or part time and either face to face or virtual. Education is provided by private companies, further education establishments, corporate businesses, dental schools, trusts and the military. All these settings require education teams and quality assurance teams, as well as members of the team who can invigilate in examinations if required. Many of the awarding bodies also have educational roles for dental nurses, which include being examiners, invigilators and presiding examiners for both the primary and postregistration awards. All of these require periods of training, competence assessing and regular updates. Each dental nurse qualification awarding body has its own requirements, but by contacting them and staying abreast of opportunities, this is another exciting career choice. This can also lead to roles such as being an external examiner or holding educational positions with the GDC, becoming a key opinion leader or an auditor.

Taking the path of the assessor or becoming part of the quality assurance team is another option in the world of dental nurse education. Both require formal training; the assessor works closely with the student and assesses their work to occupational standards. The internal quality assurer (IQA) moderates and samples the assessor's work over time and ensures standardisation of activities and decisions and approves students to reach completion. The external quality assurer monitors and overseas the roles of the assessors, IQA and the providing centres. Dental nurses can train and undertake qualifications for these role. The roles noted are currently more aligned to apprenticeship work, although the other level 3 qualifications and equivalents all have very similar roles.

Becoming a *formal mentor and/or supervisor* also requires additional training and the undertaking of a formal qualification is recommended. The role requires individuals to act within an ethical framework and code of practice, which places the mentee at the heart of any activity. Once trained, it is important to maintain skills and be supervised annually, so that this is part of the mentor's annual CPD. There are many forms of mentoring – not all are formal but working within predetermined parameters is essential to enable a trusting yet professional relationship to develop. Being a mentor does sometimes stray into being a coach and whilst they have similarities, they are quite different. Having mentoring skills is an advantage in becoming a supervisor too, as the skills combined can be most helpful in motivating and moving mentees and students forward. Qualifications and training are available at all levels; they are not specific to dentistry but then, the need is not specific to dentistry. Undertaking these roles adds to key transferable skill sets.

A number of dental nurses have shown an interest in being a *first aider* and have undergone training to not only teach first aid but to be relied upon in an emergency. This clearly requires extensive training and comes with clear parameters of roles and responsibilities. This is a skill set normally taught away from the dental setting and these are vital and important skills. It is important to consult both the scope of practice and the indemnity teams when undertaking these duties as a dental care professional. It may be that when applied in a different setting and under different circumstances, the scope may be different. Always be clear in what capacity you are acting and that the patient's best interests come first. First aider courses are widely available and offer transferable skills, as well as being an asset in any dental setting.

Mental health lead An invaluable role and a new one to the dental setting, which has really evolved at speed as a result of the pandemic. The role involves a stepped approach to learning and applying the skills. The purpose of the role is early intervention and safe signposting; it involves embedding mental health awareness in the workplace, through policy, at induction, in appraisal and staff meetings and training days and supporting people in returning to work. Whilst the whole team is engaged in stress awareness, the framework requires a lead or leads, depending on the size of the business, to step forward and train as a mental health first aider. The dental nursing team may be best placed to do this and again this is another rewarding role with transferable skills.

Clinic co-ordinator Another new role in the primary care setting, but an established role in the secondary care setting. This role is one that currently works well in large practices with multiple surgeries and clinicians. It involves managing clinicians' diaries, organising appointments, linking to laboratories, handling general enquiries, stock control and managing professional meetings. This role is suited to someone with high-level organisational and administrative skills who can multitask and use their initiative. Whilst predominantly in the private setting in dentistry, the role does exist in the hospital setting but tends to be a general role rather than specific to dentistry.

Other opportunities

Oral healthcare educators

Dental nurses are working in care homes supporting carers with mouth care and delivering oral care in hospital settings as part of programmes such as Mouthcare Matters and Mini Mouthcare Matters and have also been involved in dental nurse-led clinics and as part of multidisciplinary teams for head and neck cancer patients. These dental nurses are heavily involved in the patient journey from start to finish. There are a number of dental nurses who are actively involved in the Mouth Cancer Foundation charity, one is a former member of the UK Oral Management in Cancer Care Group (UKOMiC) charity (http://ukomic.com/). This charity supports people going through head and neck cancers and oral cancers, undertakes research and produces clear and succinct resources for the profession and for those undergoing treatment.

Regulatory and Royal College roles

Other than taking an employed role with these organisations, there are other opportunities as recognised dental professionals, including roles on panels and stakeholder groups and associate roles, which are remunerated on a sessional basis. Previously this was alluded to in the education section, but it applies to the GDC Fitness to Practise work and other areas. For example, an education associate is a quality assurance role reviewing providers of dental education across all categories of dental professional. Also, there are registration assessment panellists, reviewing applications for GDC registration from overseas dental professionals. These two roles are remunerated. Quite often, there are opportunities to represent professional groups at stakeholder meetings if you are a member of your professional society or association. From time to time specialist interest panels look for people too. Roles with other awarding bodies include paid roles such as a Care Quality Commission inspector.

The Royal Colleges are another source of interest. They have a number of panels and advisory boards who look for interested parties; these roles are advertised on their websites and are usually in keeping with key areas of interest, such as education and training.

An obvious choice for those taking an educational path is the Royal College of Surgeons Edinburgh, which has a Faculty of Dental Trainers. Here dental nurse educators can apply for one of the three levels: Associate, Member or Fellow, aligned to the level of experience and qualifications gained and yes, as a dental nurse like Fiona, you can gain the highest level of recognition, the Fellowship.

Hospital and secondary care settings

These workspaces combine dentistry and hospital-level care. The treatment is often complex and advanced and requires a higher level of patient care and input. Patients who have complex medical needs are most frequently seen in the hospital setting so that the appropriate dental and medical attention can be provided. This does mean that dental nurses working within these settings will need to undertake additional and specific training. Dental nurses also have the opportunity to work in multidisciplinary and interdisciplinary teams and quite often work with some of the most vulnerable patients. Many dental nurses working in this setting undertook additional training and were redeployed in the COVID-19 pandemic and others were working in critical care providing oral care (NHS 2020). These roles also extend in some cases to secure setting services, that is the prison services. These roles are frequently advertised but highly sought after. In general terms, holding the primary dental nursing qualification is the required starting point.

When it comes to opportunities to progress as a dental nurse in this area, an example from a dental school is provided in Figure 5.4.

Dental schools are secondary provider environments. In addition to the training of dental professionals, they also provide patient care,

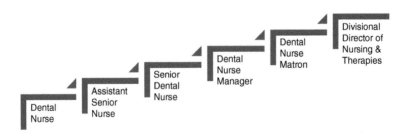

Figure 5.4 Career progression within a dental school.

including specialist areas of dentistry. Dental nurses working in dental schools have the opportunity to assist in advanced dental interventions as well as progressing along management and leadership pathways should they choose to do so.

Dental nurses are supported to undertake postregistration qualifications, and assistant senior dental nurses are supported to complete Institute of Leadership & Management (ILM) courses at level 3 as a minimum. Senior dental nurses are supported to study at level 5. There is also a pathway for dental nurses to undertake teaching and assessing qualifications. Moving through these progressive roles takes time and in certain cases there are requirements to have been in a role for a number of years and have a broad level of experience across dentistry. Many of these roles require excellent interpersonal and leadership skills and are best served by individuals who wish to follow a management and more strategic pathway.

Dental nurses in the military

Dental nurses can enter the military as a registered dental nurse or train after entry to become a dental nurse. Dental nurses can also become reservists or engage in the civilian workforce. All three military services have their own specific entry criteria. This section gives a brief overview of the entry requirements and progression opportunities.

Royal Navy (2022)

Invites applicants to an initial presentation, followed by a defence aptitude test and an interview with the medical recruiting team. Next there is an attestation phase and a medical and fitness test with the need to pass the naval swimming test. You then spend time learning about life at sea and are required to undertake a weapons course. Once early training is successfully completed, dental nurses become part of the medical branch. The role includes providing support to military operations at sea, on land and in the air. First promotions are to Leading Hand and second promotion is to Petty Officer based upon merit.

Royal Air Force (2022)

Dental nurses can join as full-time regular recruits or as spare time reserves and can apply to join as a registered dental nurse or a student dental nurse. Applicants must meet the health and fitness criteria and pass the defence aptitude test. You are expected to provide high-level care in the UK and overseas and you will be taught military skills, weapon handling and fieldcraft. You initially join for 12 years as a full-time applicant and after one year apply to become a Senior Aircraftman/woman. With additional training, you are awarded the Technical Discriminator badge and competitive promotion to Corporal is possible. When the level of Corporal is reached, you can become a practice supervisor in the regional dental headquarters or a dental nurse instructor. Progression is very much through rank and not through dental nursing.

British Army (2022)
Applicants can join as a priority, a regular or a reservist; dental nurses can be registrants or intending to train. Fitness and medical tests are a requirement and you are taught the skills to become a soldier, including handling a rifle and fieldcraft. As a dental nurse, you are given the opportunity to undertake a number of additional duties. Rank progression is an option and other related roles are available. According to Chance (2011), as with the other military groups, there is the opportunity to undertake further qualifications. An example of this is shown below.

- First-line management.
- Intermediate practice manager.
- Managing Civilian Certificate.
- Defence trainer supervisor.
- Defence Train the trainer (staff and instructor).
- TRIM Practitioner (Trauma Risk Management - for secondary PTSD prevention).
- IOSH Certificate (Institute of Occupational Safety and Health)

It is important to note that undertaking the required weapons course provides an opportunity to gain the skills needed to protect the patient and self in accordance with the Geneva Convention (American Red Cross 2011).

'*Expect the unexpected.*' Morrison (2016) mentions another aspect of dental nursing in the military: providing dental treatment and care for attack and search dogs. Without this care, the dogs would be stood down and a loss to the mission. It is not unheard of to carry out endodontic and crown treatments or be involved in trauma work with military dogs (Ministry of Defence 2013). Oral health for military dogs is essential as they are key members of the working team and how many dental nurses get to be part of contemporary dentistry for animals?

Dental nurses within the military are very much involved in ensuring that all personnel have dental fitness and as far as reasonably possible, that the risk of dental disease-causing issues whilst out in the field or dental emergencies occurring is vastly reduced. The teams predominantly provide care and support to military personnel and their families. In unique situations such as war zones, the military provide oral care through the community services. The military are an example of where the clinical role of dental nursing is combined with that of armed service. A dental nurse here would have an opportunity to learn leadership and other skills.

Examples of career pathways

As dental nursing duties are undertaken across several different settings, the following three examples provide an overview of some dental nurse career progressions. It must be noted that there are many variations of these pathways.

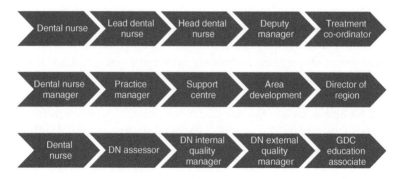

Given the wide variations of roles and settings, it is clear to see why dental nurses need to be inquisitive and creative when it comes to career planning, as it is far from straightforward. Another dimension is the dental setting, given that different types of dental care are likely to be provided in different settings and with varying team members and allied teams in some cases. These settings have in part

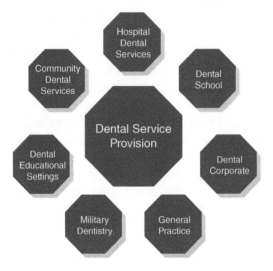

Figure 5.5 Dental settings.

been mentioned throughout the book, but here they are considered together (Figure 5.5).

In brief, hospital settings often provide more complex and challenging treatments and quite often see the most vulnerable of patients, with complex health conditions and special care needs. Those who have a keen interest in oral and maxillofacial surgery, trauma, paediatrics, orthodontics and orthognathic surgery, to name but a few, should be looking at hospital and acute settings. Those interested in dental training schools and following fields such as periodontology, dental public health and restorative work will be best suited to the dental school setting, which often form part of a university. The majority of specialists are associated within these settings.

Those with an interest in working in a referral centre, and particularly with patients who cannot be treated in general practice but do not need hospital care, would find working in the Community Dental Services (CDS) a favourable choice. The CDS also provides dental treatments in secure (prison) settings.

The largest number of dental nurses work in the primary care setting supporting general dentists and often dental therapists and hygienists. General dental practices can be private, mixed or NHS.

General treatments are provided in this setting, also minor oral surgery, implants, tooth extraction and simple orthodontics.

Other areas of interest to dental nurses include forensic odontology, Mouthcare Matters and Mini Mouthcare Matters, dental radiography, cognitive behaviour therapy and dental phobia. It goes without saying that there are rewarding experiences available for dental nurses wishing to work with vulnerable groups through the dental charities. Many of the charities not only work in developing countries, but they provide treatment and care in the UK too. Much of this work is undertaken in mobile dental units. The overseas work is reliant on having registered volunteers and being able to transport the equipment. The teams provide care in prisons, orphanages, refugee camps, slum areas and remote villages. What is important on these trips is the need to leave sustainable care behind and dental nurses with an oral health qualification have a huge part to play in this aspect of volunteering. This is about giving back and making a difference – volunteering for dental charities can provide opportunities to meet and connect with new people, gain knowledge of other ways of life and life priorities, find a sense of purpose and boost your self-confidence. It can also make for excellent conversations in interviews and could improve job prospects.

There have been further career developments since mandatory registration, one of the most prominent being agency and freelance working. More and more dental nurses are turning to these ways of working, because they offer more flexible modes of working, variety and greater opportunities to utilise and maintain skills, and attract higher salaries. Without doubt, this is impacting upon the current vacancies in dental nursing across the UK and informing new workforce trends.

Another prominent career development has been the rise of private enterprises providing not only primary education but also postcertification and CPD courses. CPD provision has certainly seen the rise of the dental entrepreneur.

Finally, it is pertinent to mention the arm of the dental trade workforce. As dental nurses have gained more knowledge and experience and developed self-confidence, more are finding roles within the dental trade environment, where they can combine their dental interests with dental sales.

For some people dental nursing can be a gateway to other healthcare and social care careers, This was particularly noticeable during the COVID-19 pandemic when dental nurses stepped up. The skill transfer demonstrated was remarkable. In times of crisis when needs must, there will always be individuals who take opportunities to grow and change.

It is easy to see why there needs to be a commitment to career decision making and a readiness to address career problem solving. Having given a whistle stop tour of opportunities within dentistry and the roles that dental nurses can undertake, it makes sense now to look at how to build your career.

Shape of your career

Each career is unique. The shape of your career is also unique alongside the individual components within it. You may like to ponder two shapes: the climbing frame and the ladder. The climbing frame represented in Figure 5.6 by a children's playground depicts a career that has many different components, but no one fixed direction. This type of career fits well with portfolio working. In contrast, there is the ladder shape (Figure 5.7) which represents a career that travels in one direction towards a goal, which has been the more traditional career shape until relatively recently. Always remember, the shape of your career is unique to you.

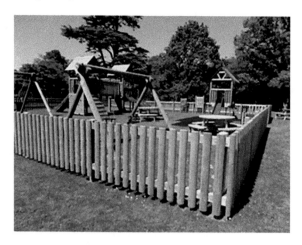

Figure 5.6 Climbing frame.

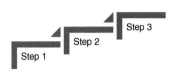

Figure 5.7 The ladder.

Developing a professional portfolio

The professional portfolio is a comprehensive collection of examples of evidence that demonstrate your experiences, capabilities and employment potential. Professional portfolios can demonstrate that as a dental nurse you are self-reflective, proactive and engaged in the development process. Before embarking upon developing a professional portfolio, always ask yourself what is its purpose?

Professional portfolios can be developed as a digital resource or a physical resource. Whichever format you prefer, it is ideal to keep all the evidence in one place. There are no hard and fast rules on what a professional portfolio should look like, but the following list has been provided as a point of reference.

- Cover page
- Table of contents
- Resumé – a personal statement with an overview of your career, inspirations and career goals
- Core curriculum vitae
- Letters of recommendation and, where possible, references
- Evidence – awards, certificates, photos
- Any research outlines and publications
- Record of CPD and any career learning plans
- Professional goals
- Volunteering work

Professional portfolios are utilised across a number of professional disciplines and are a way of seeing professional growth and development over time; they are also a reflective instrument. Clark and Eynon (2009) summarise the professional portfolio as a means of collecting, selecting, reflecting and connecting through delivery of a portfolio.

Curriculum vitae design

Oermann (2002) asserts that the professional portfolio helps individuals 'market themselves when applying for career ladder positions or new jobs'. A crucial part of your portfolio is your curriculum vitae (CV). We recommend that you keep both a 'core' CV, which includes your main achievements, but also a 'resource' CV which includes all your achievements. The core CV is part of your portfolio whilst the resource CV is only for your use. This is the document that you will use when preparing to apply for a new role or position. It means you won't forget anything you have accomplished so far, which is easier to do than you may think, particularly if you have been working for a few years.

When you apply for a new role, tailor your CV to that role and that organisation or practice; do not use the core CV. Your tailored CV and an application form (if one is used) are the documents that get you an interview. It is well worth spending time building both your resource CV and your portfolio. Do this when you have time to think and reflect back over what you have achieved rather than when you are looking for new posts. Sometimes a new post comes up at short notice when you are least expecting it. If you have your resource CV, you can quickly put together a CV for this new opportunity.

Your resource CV will grow and you should review it regularly, adding new things you have completed. These can be projects you have undertaken, new responsibilities you have taken on, new training you have completed. Don't forget what you do outside the surgery/practice. Many voluntary roles demonstrate skills that are transferable back into dentistry. If you are unsure how to start building your CV, it can be worth working with a mentor to ensure it is the best it can be.

Promoting yourself

An enthusiastic colleague who is eager to learn and develop themselves is usually much more in demand than one who just turns up. If you really want to get on, this will show and you are much more likely to find that opportunities come your way. Be the dental nurse who is curious and inquisitive. Be the dental nurse who steps up and joins in.

Dentistry can be isolating, as we often work in small units with a small number of colleagues. Widening your focus helps other people to get to know you and your skills. Whenever you can, get along to activities outside the practice, join a dental nurse professional group, take part in what is on offer. This broadens your knowledge about what is happening and increases your network of colleagues.

Show that you are a dental nurse who is competent, capable and wants to grow. This is all part of promoting yourself in a good way and developing your own personal brand and professional identity.

References

American Red Cross (2011). Summary of the Geneva Conventions of 1949 and Their Additional Protocols. Available at: www.redcross.org/content/dam/redcross/atg/PDF_s/International_Services/International_Humanitarian_Law/IHL_SummaryGenevaConv.pdf

Arthur, M., Khapova, S., Wilderom, C. (2005). Career success in a boundaryless career world. *Journal of Organizational Behavior*, **26**, 177–202.

British Army (2022). Dental Nurse Army Medical Service. Available at: https://apply.army.mod.uk/roles/army-medical-service/dental-nurse

Brown, D., Brooks, L. (2002). *Career Choice and Development*, 4th edn. Jossey-Bass, San Francisco.

Chance, S. (2011). An opportunity that didn't happen by Chance. Available at:www.dental-nursing.co.uk/news/an-opportunity-that-didnt-happen-by-chance

Clark, J.E., Eynon, B. (2009). E-Portfolios at 2.0 – surveying the field. Available at: https://go.gale.com/ps/i.do?id=GALE%7CA205052193&sid=googleScholar&v=2.1&it=r&linkaccess=abs&issn=15411389&p=AONE&sw=w&userGroupName=anon%7Ebf13c19a

Horton, L. (2010) Implementing a treatment coordinator in your practice. Available at: www.horton-consulting.com/wp-content/uploads/2018/07/aug2010.pdf

Mercer, P., Bailey, H., Cook, P. (2007). Perceptions, attitudes and opinions of general dental practitioners and dental nurses to the provision of lifelong learning for the dental team. *British Dental Journal*, **202**, 747–753.

Ministry of Defence (2013). RAF dentist treats military working dog. Available at: www.gov.uk/government/news/raf-dentist-treats-military-working-dog

Morrison, J.P. (2016) Expect the unexpected. Available at: www.dental-nursing.co.uk/features/expect-the-unexpected-1

National Health Service (NHS) (2020). Redeploying the clinical dental work-force to support the NHS clinical delivery plan for COVID-19. Available at:www.england.nhs.uk/coronavirus/documents/redeploying-the-clinical-dental-workforce-to-support-the-nhs-clinical-delivery-plan-for-covid-19/

NICE (2015). Oral Health Promotion: general dental practice (NG30). Available at: www.nice.org.uk/guidance/ng30

Oermann, M.H. (2002). Developing a professional portfolio in nursing. *Orthopaedic Nursing*, **21**(2), 73–78.

Office for Health Improvement and Disparities (2021). Delivering Better Oral Health. Available at: www.gov.uk/government/publications/delivering-better-oral-health-an-evidence-based-toolkit-for-prevention

Osborn, A.F. (1953). *Applied Imagination: Principles and Procedures of Creative Thinking*, 3rd edn. Charles Scribner's Sons, New York.

Perkins, A. (2019). Describing your professional journey – a simple 3-part script. Available at: www.anitaperkinsconsulting.com

Ross, M.K., Ibbetson, R.J. (2006). Educational needs and employment status of Scottish dental nurses. *British Dental Journal*, **201**, 661–666.

Royal Navy Dental Nurse Careers (2022). Available at: www.royalnavy.mod.uk/careers/roles-and-specialisations/services/surface-fleet/dental-nurse

Royal Airforce Dental Nurse Recruitment (2022). Available at: https://recruitment.raf.mod.uk/roles/roles-finder/medical-and-medical-support/dental-nurse

Shockley, M.K., Ureksoy, H., Rodopman, O.B., Poteat, L.F., Dullaghan, T.R. (2016) Development of a new scale to measure subjective career success: a mixed-methods study. *Journal of Organizational Behavior*, **37**, 128–153.

Chapter 6 **The future**

The profession of dental nursing is still evolving both proactively and reactively. As dental nurses step up and become agents for change within the profession, prospects can be both exciting and daunting. This chapter will scan the future for dental nursing and dental nurses.

We're going to stick our necks out and say that we think the future for dental nursing is bright. There is still a lot to do and scientific and technological discoveries will have a big impact on dentistry, both in the profession and how services (and what services) are delivered. Those in dentistry really must become more engaged in the bigger picture both inside and outside the profession.

It is surely safe to assume that for the dental nurses who qualify in 2023, their careers will be very different from dental nurses who are about to retire. This does not mean the contract, it means maybe practising on the moon base or the Mars base – it means thinking so far outside the box, there is no box.

In the introductory chapter we noted the considerable changes that have occurred over our own careers, some predictable, many not and a few almost mystical. In 1979, mobile communications were unheard of and now it is almost impossible to conduct our lives without the latest mobile phone. Of course, the last thing that we do is use our phones to call anyone. These are mobile devices by which we conduct our lives and our business. Dental practices must be connected, must have websites. The information technology revolution has been just that – science fiction became science fact.

The demands placed upon the dental workforce have never been higher and with an eye on integrated care systems and beyond, it is important that the profession is geared up to providing a system that is both agile and accepting of such change. This means finding the

How to Develop Your Career in Dental Nursing, First Edition. Edited by
Janine Brooks and Fiona Ellwood.
© 2023 John Wiley & Sons Ltd. Published 2023 by John Wiley & Sons Ltd.

construct between dental nurses, career pathways and the capacity to transition from primary qualification seamlessly to a career of choice and one of purpose. This goes beyond 'scaling up' to meet a service need – this is about being courageous and creative and rethinking, it is time to modernise the dental nursing career world.

The future of dental nursing and the future of dentistry clearly go hand in hand. Dentistry is itself intrinsically bound to the wider world. As we consider what the future holds for dental nurses and dental nursing, we need to link this with an exploration of how dentistry itself will evolve in our highly scientific, highly technical world. Dentistry is affected by advances in medical science and will adapt in ways that we may be able to predict but also in ways that today we cannot even imagine. In addition, it will be important to consider the profession of dental nursing but also the individual dental nurse.

The scene is set for three major threads: dentistry; the profession of dental nursing and the individual dental nurse, all intrinsically linked but also separate. We will review some of the factors that are likely to impact on each of these threads, plus give our own take on how each thread might respond to futures that could become a reality. We will largely postulate but hopefully with a large dose of reality. But before we think about dentistry, we have to think about the wider environment, the world outside dentistry.

The world outside dentistry

Dentistry does not operate in a vacuum. We are part of healthcare. We are part of the wider scientific world, the wider technological world, the wider philosophical world. Advances and developments outside dentistry may not always affect how we operate but frequently they do and not always as we might be able to predict. Changes in society also impact on the profession and the provision of service. Very often, those who work within dentistry have little influence on these advances and developments – think about the worldwide web, mobile telephones, email. These amazing developments came from outside dentistry but they have had a massive impact on how we educate students, how we undertake CPD, how we communicate with each other and our patients. The world changes around us and we need to adapt to it.

Here are a few current advancements that are with us now. Think about stem cell therapy and the revolution that will bring for tooth replacement. Think about virtual reality and how that is changing the way dental professionals are educated. Think about digital technology and how that has affected how we make our records and communicate with our patients. Many recent advances are being refined and their full potential is yet to be revealed, but all are likely to affect dentistry in the not so distant future – some already do. We don't know what we don't know, so we can only speculate about advances still to be made. When Fiona and I qualified, we had no conception of how viral infections would affect how we worked, the need for gloves, masks, better decontamination, these were just around the corner for us.

A small illustration of how fast the future becomes the present and then becomes the past can be seen in our own careers which span over 40 years from entering training to the present day. Figure 6.1 traces some of the incredible advances that have occurred since the late 1970s. Most of them have affected dentistry but all have impacted on our personal lives. Looking back, it's been a rollercoaster ride of massive change. And this is not a rollercoaster that will stop or slow down – it's exciting and terrifying in equal measure.

We have included just a small number of the advances we have witnessed during our working careers. Others we could have added are holographic technology, i-pads, web TV, autonomous vehicles, bionic limb advancement, smart pills, surgical superglue, smart contact lenses and many more. I'm sure you get the point we are making – the technological advances are dazzling. It's also worth thinking about the pace of technological advancement – it seems to be speeding up (and up).

Dentistry is notoriously focused, some might say isolated, in its thinking. Unless something has dentistry written in large flashing lights, some in the profession just don't register what they read about as being important to dentistry. For example, mRNA vaccines will revolutionise the treatment of head and neck cancers. Table 6.1 notes just a few more developments that will change dentistry and those who work in the profession beyond recognition in the near future. There will be many other incredible developments that we can't even imagine today. How can we prepare ourselves for what we are not aware of and what is still to be discovered? A growth mindset will be a considerable asset, combined with flexibility and a willingness to

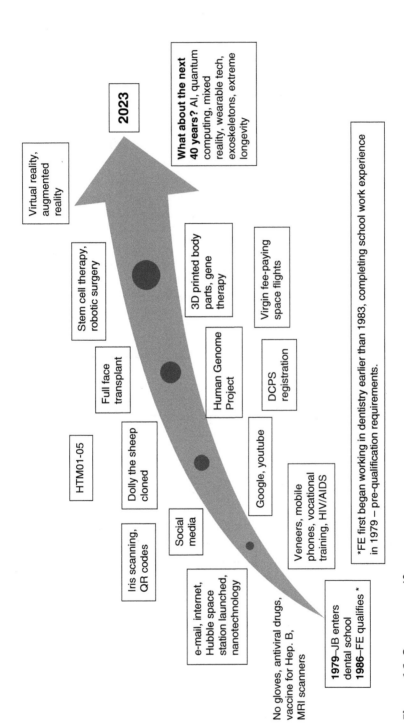

Figure 6.1 Our careers – 40 years.

Table 6.1 Technological advances (a few).

Tele-dentistry	Human Genome Project	Space – the final frontier	CRISPR – gene editing
Metaverse	mRNA vaccines	Artificial intelligence and machine learning	Wearable data
Stem cell technology	Gene therapy and editing	Digital health	Health sensors
3D printing	Smart toothbrushes	Virtual consultations	Robotics
Virtual reality learning	Nanotechnology	Mixed reality	

re-evaluate and adapt. The knowledge that life-long learning is crucial and retraining is a certainty, as old techniques and roles diminish and new ones rise to the fore. Implants may fall to stem cell technology.

Stem cell technology is an area that has massive potential. Shilpa et al. (2013) report that:

> 'Currently dental stem cell research focuses on regeneration of dentine, pulp and teeth; alveolar bone; regeneration of periodontal ligament after periodontal disease; salivary gland regeneration after radiation therapy; repair of craniofacial defects; and in the treatment of lichen planus.'

This paper is now over seven years old. The authors gave a glimpse into the future as they saw it for stem cell research and suggested:

> 'With the advances in the stem cell biology, years from now dental stem cells will hopefully be able to correct cleft palate, save injured teeth and jaw bones, correct periodontal defects, and most strikingly regenerate the entire teeth structures.'

This one advance is so exciting for dentistry and patients.

In Chapter 3 we made brief reference to the most recent advancement in Texas, whereby dental nurses are able to undertake specific duties relating to teledentistry. It is pleasing to see that guidance is unfolding to support this work as increasingly we not only turn to economical and more efficient ways of working, but we try to incorporate sustainable ethical practice and consider planetary health. Although momentum is still gathering and a number of prominent authors are now able to publish their work, teledentistry is perhaps only the start of rethinking the service provision, the end goal being to contribute to reducing the carbon footprint.

Pearl Systems are marketing 'the first comprehensive AI-powered real-time radiologic platform that automatically detects numerous conditions in dental radiographs giving dentists a second set of eyes to instantly validate radiologic findings' (www.hellopearl.com).

Hwang et al. (2019) have designed catalytic antimicrobial robots (CARs) that can controllably, effectively and accurately remove, degrade and kill biofilm from surfaces. These systems could be used in dentistry to fight biofilm in the mouth and could change the way we deal with periodontal disease forever.

Mixed reality is an exciting prospect for both clinical procedures and education of students. As described by Blanchard et al. (2022), this is a step beyond augmented reality, blending the physical world with the digital world. This technology also has the potential to enhance the consent process, helping patients to increase their understanding of complex treatments.

New technology may not be all good for manpower in dentistry. A study at Oxford University by Cheema and Dhillon (2012) found that tasks undertaken by dental hygienists and dental nurses were more likely to be replaceable by robotics than the tasks of dentists. Also, 'the use of robotics in dental clinics especially in the tasks of dental assistants may constitute one of the most important arguments for robotic dentistry'.

The small number of examples above are already in the present rather than the future, but they point the way to a future that will make dentistry very different and probably unrecognisable to dental professionals trained solely in the dental 'arts'. The future is exciting, mind-boggling and potentially scary. What is known is that dentistry will change dramatically and those who continue to work within it will need to be flexible and adaptable. The future will not stop coming, we need to embrace it or be relegated to the 'Jurassic Park' of dentistry.

Exciting times lie ahead for dental nurses as we embrace modernity in technology, but we must never lose sight of putting the patient's best interest first.

The future of dentistry

The future of dentistry seems to be experiencing huge change both from the way in which society and our patients pay for the service and also in what that service actually is. The way in which dentistry is delivered to patients continues to move rapidly away from individual dentist-owned practices to large corporate organisations with non-clinical stakeholder influence. There are opportunities here twinned with threats. The opportunities include practice ownership for dental nurses. The threats include reduction in autonomy of clinicians (Figure 6.2).

The practice of dentistry has also undergone considerable changes, particularly in the last 15–25 years with the rise in aesthetic and cosmetic procedures. Consumer demand for cosmetic procedures has shown an almost unprecedented thirst for dermal fillers, Botox®, tooth whitening and other beauty-enhancing procedures. Many dentists

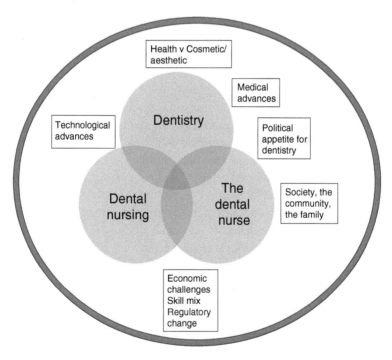

Figure 6.2 Future impacts across dentistry.

have risen to this demand. Smile clinics and dental spas have sprung up in almost every town and city in the UK. This consumer-driven change is unlikely to abate. Currently there is little or no regulation on the provision of facial aesthetics and a dental nurse who undertakes the correct training courses could begin their own business in this field.

Dental tourism, where patients travel overseas for dental procedures, has certainly increased in popularity with the public. This has brought its own challenges should problems develop once the patient returns home.

The future of dentistry can be divided into developments that are largely specific to dentistry and those that occur outside dentistry but impact on delivery, development and practice.

Taking dentistry first, where might the profession be headed in the next 20–40? It seems likely that periodontal disease will remain a challenge, whilst prosthetics is on the wane. Dental caries for most of the population is reducing although there will probably be sectors of society that are still prone to the effects of excess sugar. Dental materials continue to develop and revolutionise treatment.

Probably the greatest challenge for the oral health of the UK population for years to come is the way in which dentistry is paid for. It seems that NHS dentistry will continue to be in crisis and more patients and professionals will transition to privately funded provision. This could have the biggest effect on oral health and divide the population into those who can afford and choose to benefit from the latest techniques and those who lack motivation or the means (or both) to maintain good oral health.

Corporate dentistry continues to take a larger and larger share of dental provision with independent practice reducing year on year. This will impact on the dental professionals working within corporate dentistry as well as the patients receiving care.

Specialisation is unlikely to reduce and the future may bring more dental professionals growing their skills in specific areas with a reduction of generalists.

The rise of cosmetic and aesthetic procedures shows no sign of abating. The public have developed a thirst for looking good and celebrity culture may play a part here. Tooth whitening, adult orthodontics, dermal fillers, Botox and other facial procedures have risen in popularity. Health dentistry certainly seems to have taken a back seat with many patients. In the future, public demand may be the driver for dentistry budding off this aspect of provision.

The political appetite to continue to fund dentistry within the NHS is likely to be a major influence on the provision of dentistry as we progress. Many dentists and therefore dental nurses are moving away from NHS contracts into the private sector.

Turning to more general medical, scientific and technological advances that will impact on dentistry, these are many and exciting. Their actual effect on dentistry is hard to predict with accuracy, but it is beyond doubt that impact will be felt. An example of a new technology that has had a profound impact on dentistry is 3D printing.

The profession of dental nursing

At the beginning of the chapter it was noted that the practice of dentistry and the profession of dental nursing go hand in hand. In the UK, it is expected that a dentist will work with a dental nurse. This is less so for other clinical dental professionals, the dental hygienist or the dental therapist, but the clinical case for doing so is obvious. The practice of solo working for dental hygienists and dental therapists is largely led by economic considerations of employers. However, the point is that dental nursing as a profession closely mirrors the development of dentistry and dental services.

The future is ripe for the profession of dental nursing to expand responsibilities both clinically and non-clinically. Some examples include screening, prevention clinics, oral health training for allied professionals, smoking cessation clinics, designing and managing training, leadership.

As we look at the future landscape of dental nursing and the dental nurse, the impossible may no longer be impossible. However, a certainty is the need to have a creative and ambitious education system that supports this, one that can be agile, adaptable and flexible to adapt at pace, which perhaps currently seems like a tall order.

In Chapter 2 reference was made to the COVID-19 pandemic and the challenges that this posed. Education was forced to change at pace and mitigations agreed and applied, but this was perhaps the motivation the profession needed to embrace the field of technological developments and digital connective technologies.

The role of the instructor is almost unrecognisable and is representative of the designer of learning, someone who delivers and sets context, a resource provider and someone who facilitates the development of higher-level skills. Is this the time that learners become partners in their education and become involved in the co-design of their learning journey? Are we witnessing a shift from learning within bricks and mortar to online portals and assessments that are based upon case study presentation, massive open online courses (MOOCS) and simulation?

Planetary health is also forging its way into dental nursing education and practice and along the way this is perhaps likely to be an expectation from the regulator. It is already a consideration in the medical arena. The climate crisis educational integration will need to have its champions and pioneers and there is no reason why dental nurses cannot take up this baton. Already we have seen dental nurses and assistants leading the way and presenting as part of the COP26 global oral health conference. Those dental nurses studied as part of a course designed and delivered by both Berlin and Glasgow University, gaining higher-level learning skills, the first group of dental nurses and assistants to do this. The impact is reflected within the following quote from a student.

'The experience was truly incredible, I have learned so much and it has changed the way I look at things, it has made me think on a population level rather than on a patient to patient interaction and given me an insight into what dental nurses can do. I would never have imagined I would be involved in anything like this and I would encourage dental nurses to get involved if they get the opportunity, things like this are rarely there for dental nurses to get involved with.'

Individual dental nurses

Each individual dental nurse will tread their own career path. Within dentistry there are many and varied opportunities for a dental nurse to experience, both clinical and non-clinical.

The College of General Dentistry (2022) has developed a career pathway structure for dental professionals. The structure is appropriate for all categories of dental professional. It is not based on taking examinations but it builds within a Certified Membership Scheme. The structure identifies five 'levels' of achievement as demonstrated in Figure 6.3. Each level of achievement has five domains.

- Clinical and technical – the capability to diagnose, advise and treat.
- Professionalism – the conduct and behaviour to engage patient trust and confidence.
- Reflection – awareness of personal impact, abilities and limitations.
- Development – commitment and capability to improve the service to patients.
- Agency – the ability to resolve solutions independently and through others.

The pathway has been developed to give structure and support to all members of the dental team as they progress their career. It encourages reflective practice.

At about the same time as the work being undertaken by the College of General Dentistry, the Society of British Dental Nurses was also working on career pathways. The pathway devised, as depicted in Figure 6.4, has a central focus on dental nursing and recognises that

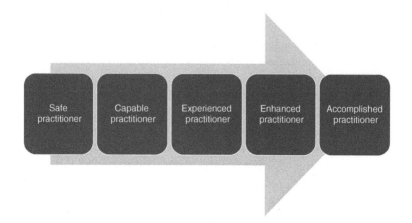

Figure 6.3 Career pathways for dental professionals. Source: College of General Dentistry 2022/College of General Dentistry.

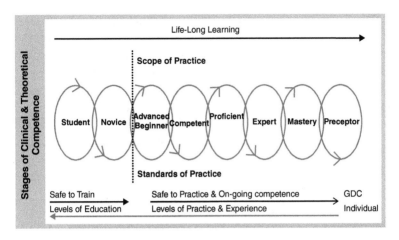

Figure 6.4 Career opportunities. Source: Society of British Dental Nurses (2021).

those who are continually learning will not necessarily always take a single trajectory. An individual dental nurse can be both an advanced beginner in one area of their work, for example undertaking an advanced skill, and an expert in another, for example charting. This will depend on the skills being learnt and demonstrated, in addition to the stage of their career. Of course, this is the case for any dental professional and the loops back and forth as we all progress should be acknowledged in any model. Figure 6.4 is also interesting in that it brings into the model pre-initial or primary qualifications, the state of being a student and novice.

Both models are helpful in their generic application for all categories of dental professional at any stage of their career.

Both models, whilst being recognised as pathways, are actually more about a direction of development than a fixed pathway with a specific goal. Unless specialist training is being undertaken, careers are more about development than pathways. One might almost suggest that pathways are twentieth entury and development (as in portfolio) is more aligned to twenty-first century thinking. Developing a variety of skills is more likely to prepare an individual for opportunities as they arise. Each of us has a unique career with unique achievements. Whilst it is interesting to look to role models and find out more about how an individual achieved a specific position, replicating their career is unlikely to be a reality.

Occasionally career development is judged by the financial remuneration attached to a post. Financial considerations are clearly important but if that is the only criterion on which a post is judged then this can very quickly lead to disappointment. Reward packages that include a wider variety of reward are most likely to be fulfilling and maintain motivation for longer. Individuals need to be valued, respected and acknowledged. Perhaps in the relatively near future standard frameworks can be agreed for terms and conditions for dental nurses.

Thoughts on future training

Initial training could be expanded to include current additional duties and strengthen skill mix and benefit patient care. This may also raise the level of the qualification to level 4. If we look back at the content and provision of dental nurse training, it can be seen that curricula and areas of learning have changed very little over the years. This is despite advancements in knowledge and techniques, as well as the evolution of technologies.

The advanced dental nurse practitioner

The future is an opportunity to introduce the advanced dental nursing practitioner. This of course will need to be supported with advanced skill training and supervision. Such a practitioner could screen patients and undertake initial medical and dental histories. The role could include devolved duties of oral health instruction and oral health promotion. In addition, smoking cessation sessions for patients and supporting patients with alcohol moderation, perhaps supporting diabetic patients and others with long-term conditions could be undertaken. It would be appropriate for an advanced dental nurse practitioner to be part of multidisciplinary teams in health settings and beyond.

Twenty-first century skills

We are now a fifth of the way through the twenty-first century and most big businesses have come to realise that the workforce need more of what has been termed 'soft' skills. Healthcare has been late to this party, even though as a service industry, serving the needs of people, you would think it would have been an early adopter. Within health-care, dentistry hasn't even been at the front of the back of the queue, so to speak.

Dentistry is a highly technical profession, interventions are our bread and butter – new materials, new techniques, new 'kit'; these are the things that underpin most dentists' daily lives. However, if that is all we invest in then we are missing the biggest trick in the book. Dentistry is highly technical, but it is also highly interpersonal. Of all the health services, dentistry has one of the most personal relation-ships with the individuals, the patients, whom we serve and from whom we make our living. We work more closely with our patients and undertake more complex procedures on a more regular basis than our other healthcare colleagues. Patients rarely can judge us on our technical, clinical skills – they trust and assume that we are com-petent and trained to perform dentistry. What they do judge us on are our 'soft' skills and patients are becoming more demanding that we are not only competent, but excel in those skills. You are judged by your chairside manner and ability to interact with your patients to a highly sophisticated degree. Dentistry is about people; the rest, which dentists think the most important, is secondary.

Many papers have been written on the type of skills and personal attributes that businesses are seeking. Eleven of the 16 'crucial profi-ciencies in the twenty-first century' identified by the World Economic Forum are non-technical.

- Communication
- Teamwork
- Problem solving
- Emotional judgement
- Professional ethics
- Critical thinking
- Creativity
- Leadership
- Entrepreneurship
- Cultural intelligence
- Digital literacy

They could have been picked with dentistry in mind. Not only are these skills deemed essential to modern workers, they are portable and transferable. We don't know what challenges dental nurses will face in their career, and still less how dentistry will change in the next 40 years. The best we can do is equip ourselves with sufficiently transferable skills to be able to respond to whatever the future holds. However, that's for the future – what about the here and now? If you want to be the best you can and to enjoy your work in dentistry then now is the time to think about investing in the sort of skills that will give you the future now.

Within dentistry, all the above skills underpin engaging with patients and bringing out the best in staff and colleagues. Almost all these skills require some level of acquisition of knowledge and training plus practice. It is rare for them to be innate although clearly some individuals are naturally gifted.

As we move forward, the need for soft skills and mentoring that can support them will only increase and intensify. Dental practices and businesses will increasingly appreciate that dental nurses with good communication skills build better relationships with patients and generate more patients as recommendations grow. Dental professionals with enhanced critical thinking and problem-solving ability will identify potential issues before they cause problems, implementing solutions early. Dental nurses who work effectively and efficiently as part of a team will develop better self-management skills and need less close oversight. Reliability will increase and sickness absence will decrease. Professionals with good emotional intelligence and deeper cultural intelligence will grow a better workforce culture, improving motivation and reducing staff turnover so that good, well-trained dental nurses are retained within the business.

The dental nurse has the potential to be so much more within the team. Figure 6.5 demonstrates the technical, personal and soft attributes that the future dental nurse should aspire to develop.

Figure 6.6 highlights a variety of impacts that will grow as we move forward into the future and that dental nurses should take account of when growing their career and thinking of how their role will develop. Most are exciting, a few could seem a little daunting. Ensuring we keep a careful watch on our own health is often forgotten until we reach a crisis point. We all play a part in keeping an eye on colleagues.

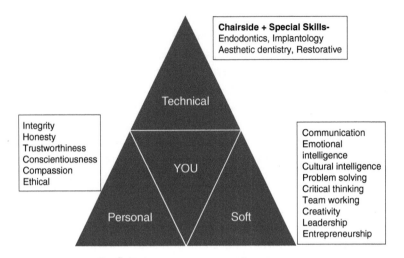

Figure 6.5 Being the full package.

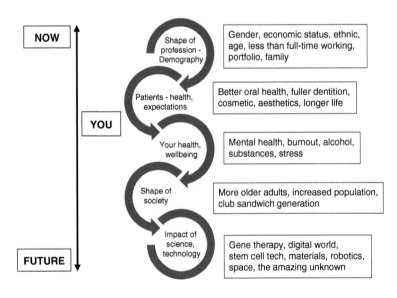

Figure 6.6 Impacts on individual dental nurses.

Examples to build your working portfolio and progress your career

Brooks (2019), in her book reviewing 100 years of women in the dental profession in the UK, included case studies of inspirational women across all categories of dental professional. Seven dental nurses are profiled. One of those dental nurses continued their career to qualify as a dental hygienist, a dental therapist and then a dentist, winning Dental Foundation trainee of the year in 2016–17, an extremely impressive individual.

Table 6.2 includes just a few of the many opportunities that exist to build a portfolio career – all can be undertaken part-time and all can be combined to shape the career you want. It takes time to build a portfolio career and it's important to try different dental environments to find those you enjoy most. Experience grows and further training and continuing professional development hone skills and knowledge. The women showcased by Brooks (2019) demonstrate the vast diversity of working niches that dental nurses occupy: workforce development; training programme delivery; author; editorial board membership; external examiner; national working party membership; divisional director of nursing (dental school); professorships; senior lecturer; coach. All began as clinical, chairside dental nurses

Table 6.2 Portfolio career ideas.

General practice	Community	Hospital	Corporate body	Military
Author	Coach	Tutor	Assessor	Mentor
Public health	Speciality	Expert witness	Dental journalist	GDC F2P panellist
Researcher	Appraiser	Politics	Development adviser	External examiner
GDC assessment panellist	GDC education associate	Treatment co-ordinator	Educationalist	Volunteer
Academic	Non-executive director	Trustee	Secure settings	GDC case worker
Internal quality assurance	Supervisor	External quality assurance		

who loved working with patients but wanted more. These dental nurses are role models for all in dentistry, not just dental nursing. The areas of working shown in Table 6.2 are given to shine a light on some aspects of dentistry you may not have considered. They include dental environments, such as general dental practice, as well as specific roles, such as a GDC fitness to practise panellist. Most need additional training and some require additional qualifications.

When we look at more current times it is apparent that there is a growing mindset and ambition to develop a unique professional identity, a narrative that once would have been alien to dental nursing. Coaching in developing such an identity relies on supporting dental nurses in defining who they are at work and what skills they bring to the workplace. The purpose of designing a professional identity is to generate and create unique opportunities that fit professional profiles. This may also reach out to the world of credentialling, celebrating and showcasing successes and skill matching for specialist roles, and the advanced dental nursing practitioner pathways to enable a broader contribution to preventive measures, dental and oral care and potentially autonomous working, leading to greater job satisfaction. It is possible for the dental nurse to demonstrate advanced clinical practice involvement, leadership and management skills, knowledge and behaviours or take part in high-level education and research. There are already a small number of dental nurses with higher degrees. There are an increasing number of dental nurses with Masters degrees and those taking doctorate paths. This may also be the dawning of acknowledging progression through the recognition of competence.

Involvement in research should grow in the future. Dental nurses are slowly pushing at research doors. There are currently research studies in which dental nurses are co-investigators and small research projects are being sponsored by dental companies. Barriers exist for all dental professionals to undertake research and the challenge is to navigate and acquire research skills. Research can begin within the dental practice; it does not have to be large scale. Skills such as critical thinking can be developed.

We must not forget the world of politics and seats at various stakeholder tables, where the voices of dental nurses have slowly started to find a place in the UK. It would be remiss to overlook those who have been awarded Queen Elizabeth II honours too, if not to simply acknowledge the fact that dental nurses continue to be recognised at the highest levels.

It is important to acknowledge that not every dental nurse wishes to progress or undertake further qualifications, but rather wants to be the best that they can be whilst undertaking a job that they love. This should not be viewed as lack of ambition or as standing still, but rather as a constant drive to be as good as you possibly can be. Dentistry and good patient care cannot exist without dental nurses who love their clinical work and who wish to continue working chairside with patients. Perhaps encouraging such dental nurses to work as champions or experts in their place of work and development of non-technical skills and advocacy for the dental nursing profession could find a place here.

So, what are our predictions for the future of dentistry over the next 100 years (if dentistry still exists, which we hope it does)?

- New technologies and scientific discoveries will change what dentistry is. For example, caries and periodontal disease will no longer be common problems. Growing teeth using stem cell technology will allow replacement of patients' lost or damaged teeth – implants, bridges, crowns and endodontics will be consigned to the history books. It is possible that these new technologies will change the need for dentistry beyond all recognition.
- Childcare, family and other carer responsibility will be shared between males and females as appropriate for the individual and their family. Society will recognise that provision of that care should not be gender dependent (or assumed).
- Values-based recruitment of dental nurse students will replace academic achievement as the prime requirement for entry to training.
- New specialties will be born, perhaps specialists in regenerative dentistry. Dental nurses will develop their clinical skills alongside dentists to work as specialist teams. Clearly this is already happening – the prediction is for new specialties.
- Portfolio careers will become the norm – either a diverse career within one working environment or across environments.
- Changing careers will become the norm – possibly requalifying in more than one career during a person's working life.
- Full-time and part-time working will no longer be relevant – the quality of hours spent will be more important.

- Training of dental professionals will radically change – 'climbing-frame' education will replace single-stream training. This type of training will open up opportunities for dental nurses who come to education late on or those who blossom academically later after leaving full-time education.
- We will no longer need to celebrate the success of women – it will be the norm for women to take each and every opportunity in dentistry, just as it will be for men.

You may think much of the above is 'pie in the sky'. Look back 100 years and try to imagine what the dental nurses of that time would make of what we have in 2023. Would they have thought modern dentistry, society, working patterns, communication technology and man walking on the moon was 'pie in the sky'? Very likely.

References

Blanchard, J., Koshal, S., Morley, S., McGurk, M. (2022). The use of mixed reality in dentistry. *British Dental Journal*, **233**(4), 261–265.

Brooks, J.A. (2019). *100 years of Women in the Dental Profession in the UK, 1918–2018*. Cambridge Scholars Publishing, Cambridge.

Cheema, H.S., Dhillon, P.K. (2012). Robotics in dentistry. *Dentimedia*, 17, 61–62.

College of General Dentistry (2022). Career Pathways in Dentistry – Professional Frameworks. Available at: https://cgdent.uk/career-pathways/

Hwang, G., Paula, A.J., Hunter, E. E., et al. (2019). Catalytic antimicrobial robots for biofilm eradication. *Science Robotics*, 4(29), eaaw2388.

Shilpa, P.S., Kaul, R., Sultana, N., Bhat, S. (2013). Stem cells: boon to dentistry and medicine. *Dental Research Journal*, **10**(2), 149–154.

Society of British Dental Nurses (2021). Career Opportunities – Dental Nursing Professional Pathway. Available at: www.sbdn.org.uk

Chapter 7 **Discussion and conclusions**

This concluding chapter will bring together the preceding chapters into a whole, bringing history up to date and looking beyond. We aim to offer conclusions and pose questions for readers to investigate for themselves.

We started by exploring the history of dental nursing, going back to a time before dentistry became the profession we know today. We have explored the growth of dental nursing and its variety of incarnations and duties. Exploration of the UK census returns gives a fascinating glimpse into the individual people who worked as dental nurses, their location, gender and marital status. We have charted the rise of education, training and qualifications, which have increased the status and value of dental nursing within society. We have reviewed the rise of professionalism. There have been many stumbles on the way and the road has often been stony, with steps forward and back. The story we have recounted developed through more modern times to bring us to what we know in the first quarter of the twenty-first century. We have also used our knowledge of current developments to look at future possibilities for dentistry, dental nursing and individual dental nurses over the coming years. Clearly, we can only horizon scan as none of us has any real idea of how the future will unfold. What we do know is that appreciating our history is the key to moving forward. If we do not learn from our history, we are doomed to repeat mistakes and fail to build on opportunities. It can be surprising how quickly important parts of history can be forgotten, even rewritten.

Early dental assistants in England appeared to undertake administrative and chaperone roles, although their exact duties are unknown. It seems this was also the case for dental assistants in North America,

How to Develop Your Career in Dental Nursing, First Edition. Edited by Janine Brooks and Fiona Ellwood.
© 2023 John Wiley & Sons Ltd. Published 2023 by John Wiley & Sons Ltd.

perhaps across the world. Freidson (1924) described dental assistants as falling into the category of auxiliary occupations, that is subordinate in authority and responsibility. This was because they derived their legitimacy from another occupation (that is, dentists) and had little prospect of becoming autonomous themselves. It is certainly true that the clinical role of dental nurses derives principally from that of the dentist, or the dental hygienist or dental therapist. However, this is beginning to change. Dental nurses are now registered professionals in their own right; they have their own responsibilities which the regulator, the GDC, holds them to. Some roles, such as oral health education and other health promotion roles, are largely autonomous. This development is very likely to continue in the future.

In the first quarter of the twentieth century we saw an expansion of the role of dental nurse into dental dresser, the first tentative steps into skill mix and developing a role that would sit beside dentists. Sadly, this was way ahead of its time and probably too close to the spectre of unqualified dentists for it to meet with approval from dentists. Early expansion of the role was curtailed by the 1921 Dentists Act and the range of work that dental nurses could undertake was reduced to chairside assisting, effectively removing the clinical role that briefly grew from the needs of patients and war. It would be many years before extended duties qualifications permitted dental nurses to expand their role. However, much of the dental dresser role was absorbed by dental hygiene.

The title and role of dental dresser was short-lived (1917–1921), a mere four years. The census return for 1921 shows 20 dental dressers, 16 women and four men. By the 1939 census return, there were three individuals described as dental dressers, all females, all working at the Public Health Department in Ipswich.

We have given an overview of dental nursing across the world, although clearly this is not comprehensive. Each country has taken a slightly different route for the development of dental nurses. Movement of individuals from country to country is not a smooth process. Whilst Britain was part of the European Economic Union, a dental nurse who qualified in one member country could work in any other member country. With the exit of the UK from Europe, those doors have closed for dental nurses from overseas who wish to work in Britain. There are processes whereby overseas qualified dental nurses can apply to be assessed individually by the GDC.

In 2023, the first dental nurse qualification will be 80 years old. For many years this was the only qualification available and many thousands of dental nurses successfully completed the NEBDN course. It is clear from Chapter 4 that since 2000, a number of alternative dental nursing qualifications have come to fruition which have provided additional opportunities for progression and development.

In the longer term, it is possible imagine that the advanced dental nurse with additional training/qualifications and competence could undertake the administration of infiltration local anaesthesia. This links to considerations in Chapter 6. Many dental nurses already have a role under supervision in conscious sedation and general sedation procedures and this may have the potential for expansion, with patient focus at the centre of the activity rather than career ladders.

Towards the end of the twentieth century, the role broadened and as we move forward, opportunities for the profession and the individual dental nurse are again looking promising. Individual dental nurses have blazed a trail and shown that dental nurses are capable and competent and have much to offer, whether that is within the clinical sphere or outside the surgery.

Dental nurses are vital to efficient and effective patient care. Dentistry is about team working, with each member playing their part and no-one standing alone. The employment of dental nurses has been shown to increase the number of patients a dentist can provide care for within a specific time frame (Widström and Eaton 2004, National Leadership and Innovation Agency for Healthcare 2012, p.27). Delegation of many technical duties to the dental nurse will allow the dentist more time for diagnosis, treatment planning and counselling of patients (Kravitz and Treasure 2007). As we move forward, dental nurses are beginning to fulfil their potential and this can only be to the benefit of all in the profession and most certainly to the benefit of patients.

A factor to consider when thinking about progression for individual dental nurses and the profession as a whole is time. An interesting study by Morris (1987) reviewed how females with successful careers in dentistry have reached their position. The study examined the career influences and actual decisions made by female dentists and aimed to increase understanding of barriers preventing women progressing in their careers. The author felt that it took about 12–25 years after qualification to achieve career success. At that time, children and a career were not perceived by the study participants to be compatible. Times have changed in the 35+ years since this study and the study did not include dental nurses. However, time served and obstacles to progression are still relevant today. Raising a family is also still an important issue.

Other achievements for UK dental nurses in recent years have been the rising recognition of mental health wellness and a right to thrive at work in addition to becoming involved in anti-racism work. The mental health wellness work has been co-chaired by a dental nurse and has been driven across all four nations. This also led to a UK dental nurse presenting on an international stage. Equally, as part of the anti-racism work, a dental nurse presented findings to the Chief Dental Officer of England steering group meetings. Such developments underpin the wide fora that dental nurses are involved with, bringing their knowledge and expertise to the table and contributing to debate and discussion.

This final chapter is a good place to ponder an interesting concept – the single story, in particular to think about the single story of dental nurses and the myths that exist. Chimamanda Ngozi Adichie (2009) presents the idea of the single story. Stories in this context are used to describe aspects of society and humanity, they are powerful and can inspire. We can often have default stories about individuals, but we should beware of the stereotype where a single story becomes the norm and is used to define a group. When this happens, an individual within the group is lost.

What is the single story of dental nurses? Could it be that dental nurses:

- work part-time?
- take career breaks to give birth and look after their children (the female ones)?
- tend not to have senior roles in dentistry?
- are not interested in career progression?
- have short dental careers?
- are not political?
- give fewer hours to their profession?
- are less committed to their profession than other categories of dental professional?
- believe they have no voice?

- have no prospects for progression?
- fear failure?
- enjoy imposter syndrome?

Is this really the single story of dental nurses? The list has a degree of familiarity, or it did. Is this just stereotypical myth?

The story of dental nursing and dental nurses cannot be reduced to a few characteristics – it is a tapestry of so many diverse and amazing individual stories. Someone cannot be defined as a single characteristic – a single story. All members of a group cannot be categorised in this way, it is sloppy and inaccurate. Each person is made up of multiple stories. How would you write the story of dental nurses? Hopefully, this book has given you food for thought. We invite you to compose your own story, post it on dental nurse forums, start a discussion.

We hope that we have demonstrated a deep respect for dental nurses as valued and professional team members throughout this book. Development and providing an environment where individuals can flourish are all too often linked to remuneration. Appropriate remuneration is important but it can hog the conversation when thinking about a comprehensive reward package. The work of Harris and Foskett-Tharby (2022) identifies pay as a stubborn problem, but one that very much sits alongside other factors, for example being valued. Perhaps the time is ripe for reward packages to be both courageous and creative.

In conclusion, this book is a celebration of what dental nurses have achieved in the 125+ years since the late nineteenth century. We hope it will add to the discussion about the huge talents that dental nurses possess and the considerable contribution they have made and are making to dentistry, the profession, patients and wider society. We hope it will become part of the contemporary history of dentistry. Perhaps even more importantly, we hope it has piqued your interest to look more deeply at the history of dental nursing and what it teaches us today and for tomorrow.

References

Adichie, C.N. (2009). Ted Talk: The single story. Available at: www.ted.com/talks/chimamanda_ngozi_adichie_the_danger_of_a_single_story?language=en

Freidson, E. (1924). Dental dressers. *Dental Surgeon*, **21**, 732.

Harris, R., Foskett-Tharby, R. (2022). From dental contract to system reform: why an incremental approach is needed. *British Dental Journal*, **233**, 377–381.

Kravitz, A.S., Treasure, E.T. (2007). Utilisation of dental auxiliaries – attitudinal review from six developed countries. *International Dental Journal*, **57**(4), 267–273.

Morris, I.R. (1987). A study into the lives of a group of successful women in dentistry. MSc in Dental Public Health, London Hospital Medical College.

National Leadership and Innovation Agency for Healthcare (2012). An analysis of the dental workforce in Wales. Available at: www.wales.nhs.uk/sitesplus/documents/829/Analysis%20of%20Dental%20Workforce%20Wales%202012%20Full%20Report.pdf

Widström, E., Eaton, K. (2004). Oral healthcare systems in the extended European Union. *Oral Health and Preventive Dentistry*, **2**(3), 155–194.

Appendix 1 **Timeline of important events in dentistry in the UK**

Date	Event
1858	Dental Hospital of London opened as the first clinical training school for dentists in the UK
1860	First licences of dental surgery were awarded by the Royal College of Surgeons of England
1878	First British Dentists Act – titles were protected but registration was not mandatory
1879	First UK Dental Register established for dentists
1880	British Dental Association founded
1897	Census in England – 116 women dentists – none held LDS
1917	Dental dressers introduced in Derbyshire and Birmingham
1919	Dental dressers introduced in Sheffield and Shropshire
1921	Dentists Act – only registered practitioners allowed to apply
1940	British Dental Nurses and Assistants Society established by Madeleine Winter, a dental nurse, and her dentist, Mr P. Grundy. This organisation has become the British Association of Dental Nurses (BADN)
1943	First dental hygienists trained by the Women's Auxiliary Air Force
1944	The first UK dental hygienists qualify
1948	NHS established
1956	Dentists Act – General Dental Council established as an independent regulator for dentistry – no longer a committee of the GMC
1957	Introduction of high-speed dental turbine
1958	Fluoride toothpaste first marketed in the UK
1960	New Cross Hospital began training dental auxiliaries

(Continued)

How to Develop Your Career in Dental Nursing, First Edition. Edited by Janine Brooks and Fiona Ellwood.
© 2023 John Wiley & Sons Ltd. Published 2023 by John Wiley & Sons Ltd.

(Continued)

Date	Event
1962	Dental auxiliaries qualified from New Cross General Hospital (50 in total – all single women)
1979	Dental auxiliary name changed to dental therapist
1984	Dentists Act
1985	Water Fluoridation Act
2002	Dental therapists permitted to work in general dental practice
2005	DCP registration with GDC
2006	New GDS NHS contract introduced
2007	First training course for orthodontic therapists opens – Leeds Dental Institute
2013	Direct access approved by GDC

Source: Adapted from Brooks, J. (2019). *100 years of Women in the Dental Profession in the UK 1918–2018*. Cambridge Scholars Publishing, Cambridge.

Index

How to Develop Your Career in Dental Nursing, First Edition. Edited by
Janine Brooks and Fiona Ellwood.
© 2023 John Wiley & Sons Ltd. Published 2023 by John Wiley & Sons Ltd.